The Daniel Fast Course

Leader's Guide

By Annette Reeder
The Biblical Nutritionist

Copyright© 2024 Designed Healthy Living,
Annette Reeder. All rights reserved.
Designed Healthy Living
Glen Allen, VA 23059
www.designedhealthyliving.com

Information contained in this Daniel Fast is educational and merely offers nutritional support. To my knowledge the FDA has not approved the Daniel Fast for any spiritual or physical benefit. This means you are putting your life in God's hands by applying Scripture to your health. Some physical diseases such as diabetes may require a consult with a doctor before altering the government designed eating plan.

No part of this publication may be reproduced, stored in a retrieval system, or transmitted in any way by any means-electronic, mechanical, photocopy, recording or otherwise-without prior permission of the copyrights holder, except as permitted by USA copyright law.

ISBN: 978-1-7376278-7-6

Table of Contents

DANIEL FAST COURSE LEADER'S GUIDE I

DANIEL FAST 1-WEEK PREPARATION SCHEDULE IV

DANIEL FAST 4-WEEK PREPARATION SCHEDULE VI

INTRODUCTION 1

WELCOME SECTION 2

BEFORE YOU START 3

TIPS FOR SUCCESS 4

7 STEPS TO A SUCCESSFUL DANIEL FAST 7

WEEK 1 11

WEEK 2 24

WEEK 3 36

RECIPES 50

Daniel Fast Course Leader's Guide

Dear Leader,

I'm grateful you're willing to lead a group through the Daniel Fast Course. I pray that your group is abundantly blessed by working through this course together. The Lord has provided many tools and resources to seek Him and be transformed into His likeness. Two of these which are very powerful tools are fasting and community. And that's what brings us to the Daniel Fast Course!

This guide is meant to go along with the course and the course workbook, helping you lead a group through the material. You'll find a suggested schedule as well as other helpful hints and recommendations. As with the recipes I share with my viewers, readers, and coaching members, take the ingredients you find helpful and add them to your menu, and leave out the ones that don't fit your tastes.

In other words, use what works for you and your group. This guide is not a dictator on how to complete the Daniel Fast Course or the fast itself. It's a set of instructions meant to help you succeed. Just as you might alter a recipe a friend shares with you, feel free to alter the instructions and ingredients in this guide.

About Fasting:

We often are led to do private fasts, as we see Jesus do right after His baptism, we indeed see Him encourage His listeners in the verse below.

> *"And when you fast, do not look gloomy like the hypocrites, for they disfigure their faces so that their fasting may be seen by others. Truly, I say to you, they have received their reward. But when you fast, anoint your head and wash your face, that your fasting may not be seen by others but by your Father who is in secret.*
> *And your Father who sees in secret will reward you." Matthew 6:6-8*

There are certainly times when we fast in solidarity, with only the Lord knowing and walking with us.

On the other hand, we also see examples in scripture of corporate fasts.

> *And in every province, wherever the king's command and his decree reached, there was great mourning among the Jews, with fasting and weeping and lamenting, and many of them lay in sackcloth and ashes. Esther 4:3*
>
> *"Go, gather all the Jews to be found in Susa, and hold a fast on my behalf, and do not eat or drink for three days, night or day. I and my young women will also fast as you do. Then I will go to the king, though it is against the law, and if I perish, I perish." Esther 4:16*
>
> *Is such the fast that I choose, a day for a person to humble himself? Is it to bow down his head like a reed, and to spread sackcloth and ashes under him? Will you call this a fast, and a day acceptable to the Lord? Isaiah 58:5*
>
> *Consecrate a fast; call a solemn assembly. Gather the elders and all the inhabitants of the land to the house of the Lord your God, and cry out to the Lord. Joel 1:14*
>
> *Blow the trumpet in Zion; consecrate a fast; call a solemn assembly. Joel 2:15*
>
> *And the people of Nineveh believed God. They called for a fast and put on sackcloth, from the greatest of them to the least of them. Jonah 3:5*
>
> *While they were worshiping the Lord and fasting, the Holy Spirit said, "Set apart for me Barnabas and Saul for the work to which I have called them." Acts 13:2*

Throughout God's Word, we see times for individual fasts, groups fasts, and nation-wide fasts. As a leader for the Daniel Fast Course, you fall into the group fast category.

It is a joyful responsibility to obey the Lord and sacrifice our fleshly desires for Him. It is also a blessed responsibility to serve in such a leadership role.

Our brothers and sisters in Christ are great help to us in the various parts of our journey with Him. We are to encourage and build each other up (1 Thes. 5:11), which most likely each person will need as they embark on and complete the Daniel Fast Course and the Daniel Fast itself.

As a leader, you will be a great encourager to your group and I hope to be an encourager to you. We're in this together and in the strength of the Lord will reap the rewards.

Annette and The Biblical Nutritionist Team

Prayer for Success:

Lord, guide me and help me to hear Your voice as I lead a group of brothers and sisters in Your name. Thank You for the tools graciously given us to draw closer to You and bring You more glory. As we discipline our flesh, fill our spirits; make us holy. Remind us who we are in You. Reveal to us more of Yourself. Give us Spirit-empowered self- control and self-discipline to follow this fast and spend more time with You. We praise and glorify Your name for the mighty works You have done, are doing, and will do. Amen.

The Daniel Fast Course focuses on helping prepare people for the fast, providing tips and tools to prepare for the fast, how to make the most of the fast, shopping tips, how to complete the fast, and how to end it well.

My recommendation is to complete the course before starting the 21-day fast. There are 7 sections, which can be done in one week, seven weeks, or anywhere in between. There are two schedules given below, one for 1 week and one for 4 weeks prior to starting the fast. Then, of course, there will be an additional 3 weeks for the fast itself. Pick the best plan for you and your group!

It's recommended that you complete the course once through yourself before leading the group.

Meetings should last 1-2 hours, depending on the size of the group and how much each person brings to share and discuss.

Course Dates: _____

Course Leader: _____

Course Members: _____   _____

_____   _____

_____   _____

_____   _____

_____   _____

Make sure all group members sign up for the course before the first meeting date!

Daniel Fast 1-Week Preparation Schedule

Advertise and have members sign up 1 month in advance of the start date.
Date to start advertising/promoting: _____

Pick a start date for the course: _____
(this will be the date of the 1st meeting)

Pick a start date for the fast - 1 week after course start date: _____
(this will be the date of the 2nd meeting)
Workbook: There is a download version of the Workbook available for students.

Week 1

Day 1: MEETING 1 - Gather the group either in person (preferable) or virtually. Have group members introduce themselves and share their desired goals for the fast. Go over schedule and answer any preliminary questions. Set aside time to pray for each other.

Day 2: Complete the *Introduction* and *Welcome* section of the workbook.

Day 3: Complete the *Before You Start* section of the workbook.

Day 4: Complete page 1 of *7 Steps to a Successful Daniel Fast* section of the workbook

Day 5: Complete page 2 of *7 Steps to a Successful Daniel Fast* section of the workbook.

Day 6: Complete page 3 of *7 Steps to a Successful Daniel Fast* section of the workbook.

Day 7: Rest Day/Prepare to start the fast the following day.

Week 2

Day 8: Day 1 of fast; Complete Week 1 Day 1 in the workbook; MEETING 2 - Gather the group either in person (preferable) or virtually. Review the course and answer questions. Set aside time to pray for each other.

Day 9: Day 2 of the Daniel Fast; Complete Week 1 Day 2 in the workbook.

Day 10: Day 3 of the Daniel Fast; Complete Week 1 Day 3 in the workbook.

Day 11: Day 4 of the Daniel Fast; Complete Week 1 Day 4 in the workbook; Check in with group members via phone or text; this is often a hard day.

Day 12: Day 5 of the Daniel Fast; Complete Week 1 Day 5 in the workbook.

Day 13: Day 6 of the Daniel Fast; Complete Week 1 Day 6 in the workbook.

Day 14: Day 7 of the Daniel Fast; Complete Week 1 Day 7 in the workbook.

Week 3

Day 15: Day 8 of the Daniel Fast; Complete Week 2 Day 1 in the workbook; MEETING 3 - Gather the group either in person (preferable) or virtually. Review the first week of fasting and answer questions. Ask members about any specific challenges they may have had and to share praises. Set aside time to pray for each other.

Day 16: Day 9 of the Daniel Fast; Complete Week 2 Day 2 in the workbook.

Day 17: Day 10 of the Daniel Fast; Complete Week 2 Day 3 in the workbook.

Day 18: Day 11 of the Daniel Fast; Complete Week 2 Day 4 in the workbook; Check in with group members via phone or text.

Day 19: Day 12 of the Daniel Fast; Complete Week 2 Day 5 in the workbook.

Day 20: Day 13 of the Daniel Fast; Complete Week 2 Day 6 in the workbook.

Day 21: Day 14 of the Daniel Fast; Complete Week 2 Day 7 in the workbook.

Week 4

Day 22: Day 15 of the Daniel Fast; Complete Week 3 Day 1 in the workbook. MEETING 4 - Gather the group either in person (preferable) or virtually. Review the second week of fasting and answer questions. Ask members about any specific challenges they may have had and to share praises. Set aside time to pray for each other.

Day 23: Day 16 of the Daniel Fast; Complete Week 3 Day 2 in the workbook.

Day 24: Day 17 of the Daniel Fast; Complete Week 3 Day 3 in the workbook.

Day 25: Day 18 of the Daniel Fast; Complete Week 3 Day 4 in the workbook.

Day 26: Day 19 of the Daniel Fast; Complete Week 3 Day 5 in the workbook; check in with members via phone or text, asking how they plan to end the fast without giving up what they gained.

Day 27: Day 20 of the Daniel Fast; Complete Week 3 Day 6 in the workbook.

Day 28: Day 21 of the Daniel Fast (LAST DAY!!!); Complete Week 3 Day 7 in the workbook.

Day 29: FINAL MEETING - Gather the group either in person (preferable) or virtually. Celebrate the successful completion of the Daniel Fast. Ask members to share praises, lessons, and revelations. Discuss continued accountability and support for healthy living. Set aside time to pray for each other.

Daniel Fast 4-Week Preparation Schedule

Advertise and have members sign up 1 month in advance of the start date.
Date to start advertising/promoting: _____

Pick a start date for the course: _____
(this will be the date of the 1st meeting)

Pick a start date for the fast - 4 weeks after course start date: _____
(this will be the date of the 5th meeting)

Week 1

MEETING 1 - Gather the group either in person (preferable) or virtually. Have group members introduce themselves and share their desired goals for the fast. Go over schedule and answer any preliminary questions. Set aside time to pray for each other.

Throughout week 1: Complete the Introduction, Welcome Section, before You Start Section, and 7 Steps to a Successful Daniel Fast Section of the Course Workbook.

Week 2

MEETING 2 - Gather the group either in person (preferable) or virtually. Go over the initial sections of the workbook. Set aside time to pray for each other.

Throughout week 2: Complete Week 1 of the Course Workbook.

Week 3

MEETING 3 - Gather the group either in person (preferable) or virtually. Go over sections 3 & 4 of the course. Set aside time to pray for each other.

Throughout week 3: Complete Week 2 of the Course Workbook.

Week 4

MEETING 4 - Gather the group either in person (preferable) or virtually. Go over sections 3 & 4 of the course. Set aside time to pray for each other.

Throughout week 4: Complete Week 3 of the Course Workbook. Set a meal plan (or use the one provided), make a grocery list, & go shopping.

Week 5

MEETING 5 (first day of the fast)- Gather the group either in person (preferable) or virtually. Review meal planning, grocery shopping, and mental preparation. Answer any questions that come up. Set aside time to pray for each other.

Throughout week 4: Days 1-7 of the Daniel Fast; Check in with group members by phone or text mid-week (or every day). Day 4 is often the most challenging. Pick a section or chapter of verses to read throughout the week as a spiritual focus during the fast. Review Course Workbook Week 1 material and fill in any remaining blanks.

Week 6

MEETING 6 - Gather the group either in person (preferable) or virtually. Review the first week of fasting and answer questions. Ask members about any specific challenges they may have had and to share praises. Set aside a time to pray for each other.

Throughout week 5: Days 8-15 of the Daniel Fast; Check in with group members by phone or text mid-week (or every day). Day 4 is often the most challenging. Pick a section or chapter of verses to read throughout the week as a spiritual focus during the fast. Review Course Workbook Week 2 material and fill in any remaining blanks.

Week 7

MEETING 7 - Gather the group either in person (preferable) or virtually. Review the second week of fasting and answer questions. Ask members about any specific challenges they may have had and to share praises. Set aside a time to pray for each other. Assign Section 7 of the course.

Throughout week 6: Days 16-21 of the Daniel Fast; Check in with group members by phone or text mid-week (or every day). Pick a section or chapter of verses to read throughout the week as a spiritual focus during the fast. Review Course Workbook Week 1 material and fill in any remaining blanks. Recommend watching/rewatching the "How to End the Daniel Fast" video.

FINAL MEETING (day after the last day of the fast)- Gather the group either in person (preferable) or virtually. Celebrate the successful completion of the Daniel Fast. Ask members to share praises, lessons, and revelations. Discuss continued accountability and support for healthy living. Set aside a time to pray for each other.

Use the following charts to fill in the dates of your course and fast.

1 Week Course - 3 Week Fast

Day:							
Week 1							
Week 2							
Week 3							
Week 4							

Final Meeting Date: _____

4 Week Course - 3 Week Fast

Day:							
Week 1							
Week 2							
Week 3							
Week 4							
Week 5							
Week 6							
Week 7							

Final Meeting Date: _____

Following is a copy of the Daniel Fast Course Workbook each member will receive. Added for you as a leader are sections for you to take notes that highlight topics you'd like to discuss or questions you'd like to ask in group sessions.

Introduction

The Daniel Fast is a dramatically different way of eating. It's a partial fast that comes with a smorgasbord of physical and spiritual benefits, and your success matters! So, in order to set you up for success, we've provided many aids for the course, including this workbook. This tool will help you keep track of progress through the Daniel Fast Course and 21-day fast journey.

Everything you need to succeed in the Daniel Fast is included in this book,

- An introduction section to help you prepare for the Daniel Fast.
- Weekly guidance, including sample menus, grocery lists, and recipes you can use.
- Devotions and journaling spaces.
- A guide to ending the Daniel Fast well.

There are 3 keys to success in any fast:

Planning

Intentionality

Purposefulness

Keep these in mind as you go through the course and checklist. The aim is to eliminate mindlessness and increase mindfulness in the areas of eating and relationship with the Lord.

You'll want to spend 1-2 weeks going through the preparation material and getting ready for your powerful, life-changing, 3-week journey.

Icons For Direction

▶ VIDEO this icon will mention a video in the course to watch. The title will be given.

📱 COURSE this item will be in the course to print or read.

🌿 See the instructions to follow.

✎ Write a prayer as you prepare for the Daniel Fast.

_____
_____
_____
_____
_____
_____
_____
_____
_____
_____
_____
_____
_____

Welcome Section

☐ ▶ Watch "A Message from Annette Reeder."

☐ 📱 Read Annette's Welcome.

☐ 📱 Read "Rhonda's Testimony: Dreading Fasting until…"

☐ 📱 Read the "Frequently Asked Questions."

☐ 🌿 Do you have additional questions? Ask on the Biblical Nutrition Academy Facebook page.

☐ ▶ Watch Bonus Video "Top 9 Spiritual Benefits."

Before You Start

☐ ▶ Watch "Best Way to Use this Course."

☐ Answer the Introductory Questions.

☐ ▶ Watch "Prepare Your Pantry and Prepare Your Heart."

☐ List some things you're going to purge from your pantry and your heart during the Daniel Fast.

Pantry	Heart
_____	_____
_____	_____
_____	_____
_____	_____
_____	_____

☐ Read "Foods to Prepare."

☐ List what foods you're going to prepare ahead of time:

_____ _____ _____
_____ _____ _____

☐ Read "Remove Temptations."

☐ Check here when you've removed the temptations from your pantry.

☐ ▶ Watch the video under "This Activity will get Your Kids Excited to Join You."

☐ Read "Testimony: Don't Eat with Your Eyes, But with Your Mind."

☐ ▶ Watch Bonus Video "Accomplish More on the Daniel Fast."

Tips for Success

Do what works for you and your lifestyle.

There are a lot of suggestions and recommendations for how to do the Daniel Fast, but not all of them are required. Get the main principles and tailor the fast for you. For example, menus and recipes are given, but they are simply resources, what's worked for some as they've embarked on the Daniel Fast. What's most important are the main principles:

- No sugar
- No processed food
- No meat or dairy
- No white grains (including white potatoes)
- A heart ready to hear from the Lord
- All the fruits, vegetables, nuts, seeds, and healthy fats (EVOO, Coconut oil, avocados, etc.) you want
- Whole grains – whole grain rice, wheat, sweat potatoes, quinoa, steel-cut oats, etc.

Don't get overwhelmed by the grocery list.

We've listed all ingredients needed for the recommended recipes, but many of these items you'll already have on hand. Grab a highlighter and mark the items on your shelves. If you don't want to write in the book, make a photocopy of the grocery list for shopping/marking. There is one each week.

If a recipe looks overwhelming, skip it, or make a big batch to use multiple times.

A soup can be eaten several days in a row and/or frozen. This is the same with several other recipes. (If a recipe measurement looks odd, it's because all recipes have been broken down into 1 or 2 servings. Feel free to make a bigger batch!) See our quick and easy Daniel Fast meal ideas for items perfect for on-the-go.

Utilize leftovers well.

If a recipe calls for ⅛ of a bell pepper, use the rest with other veggies and hummus another day or freeze what's leftover. Extra veggies are also great additions to a salad for later that day or the next day.

Eating out:

Most restaurants have salads available. You can ask them to hold the meat and cheese and/or order the side salad and ask for oil and vinegar for your dressing. (There's also almost always salt and pepper to add flavor!) Carry little bottles of oil and vinegar with you if a place you're going doesn't have that option. Also, many places have vegetarian and vegan options. Try to check these out ahead of time. You can stay true to the Daniel Fast and go out to eat! (And if there's a small slip-up or situation that doesn't work, don't give up. Keep moving forward with the rest of your fast.)

Eating at other people's houses.

This too is doable but can be a bit trickier. We want to accommodate our host(s) and don't want to hurt their feelings. However, most people will understand if you explain that you're doing a partial fast for a few weeks. They may offer to make something special for you, but don't expect it or require it. Carry your own dish of Daniel Fast friendly food to enjoy a meal with family and friends.

But I work, and often long hours.

Don't dismay! Anyone can do the Daniel Fast. The key is planning. Don't get caught unprepared and super hungry. That's a recipe for failure every time. When you have a chance to do meal prep, presumedly on the weekend, prepare snacks and easy-to-grab meals that you can always have on hand. Some examples are: little containers of nuts, an apple and nut butter, fresh cut veggies and hummus, a smoothie that's been frozen and left to thaw, a container of cut up berries or other fruit, a nut butter or nut butter and fruit spread sandwich on whole grain bread, a premade quinoa bowl or salad.

I'm the only one in my family doing the Daniel Fast.

We've had many team members and Biblical Nutrition Academy members in this situation. It takes a little extra work but is still doable. Most meals come with veggies, just roast them with olive oil and seasoning, or stir fry them in coconut oil. Make extra for you and skip the meat. Nuts and seeds are easy to add to most meals for some good protein. Family wants white potatoes? Skip those and fix yourself a sweet potato or add a piece of fruit instead. The extra work it takes to make things your family isn't eating IS SO WORTH IT! And remember, the Daniel Fast is only 21 days. You can do it!

Before You Start ~ Rhonda's Testimony

For many years, I associated fasting with people in the Bible or extreme situations. When the subject of fasting appeared in this study, I had a profound thought: "This is too hard!" Then the Holy Spirit worked in my heart and mind about fasting. He wouldn't let me alone. I had gone years without ever sensing His desire for me to fast.

As I read through the chapter on fasting, everywhere I turned, there were articles and books on fasting "jumping out" at me. Instead of dismissing these "coincidences", I prayed.

Questions came to my mind. "Was the Lord asking me to fast? Couldn't I do something else for the Lord? Was this really necessary?" I knew I did not have the willpower to fast. He spoke gently to my heart and said, "Keep your focus on Me. If you will walk with Me daily, I will give you the strength and grace of fasting."

Then He said something that took me by surprise, "Claim this expression of love, obedience and faith, as a 'done deal', now, even before you start the first day of fasting." Wow! This was too big. I was tempted to remind the Lord of my lack of self-discipline. He was asking me to trust Him during a fasting journey and submit to Him.

I really did not want to refuse His loving invitation. He wanted me to focus on Him and His power, not on me and my weakness. I fasted to please Him and to depend on Him alone each day. I went from fear of fasting to a deeper faith and freedom in Christ. The Lord faithfully has brought me through the "Daniel Fast" twice victoriously. Rhonda Sutton

Response/prayers before you start the Daniel Fast: _____

_____

_____

_____

_____

_____

_____

_____

_____

_____

_____

_____

7 Steps to a Successful Daniel Fast

☐ ▶ Watch "7 Steps to a Successful Daniel Fast" video.

☐ ✎ Fill in the blank: Daniel made up his _____.

☐ ✎ Fill out the Daniel Fast Commitment Card. (You can also print a separate card, found under "Make a Commitment.") The Commitment Card is found in the course.

☐ ✎ Fill out the 7 Steps.

    Step 1: _____

    Step 2: _____

    Step 3: _____

    Step 4: _____

    Step 5: _____

    Step 6: _____

    Step 7: _____

☐ 📱 Read "Make up Your Mind."

☐ 📱 Read Daniel 1.

☐ 📱 Read "Make a Commitment."

☐ 📱 Read "Make a Plan."

☐ ✎ Copy Daniel 10:2-3. _____

_____

_____

_____

_____

_____

_____

☐ ▶ Watch Bonus Video "What to Eat and What to Avoid"

- [ ] ✎ Write out what foods to be included and avoided.

    Foods to include: _____
    _____
    _____
    _____

    Foods to avoid: _____
    _____
    _____
    _____

- [ ] 📖 Read "Make Preparations."
- [ ] ▶ Watch Bonus Video "Shopping Tips."
- [ ] ▶ Watch Bonus Video "Shopping for Greens."
- [ ] 📋 Schedule a grocery shopping day with your Daniel Fast grocery list: _____.
- [ ] 📋 Schedule a meal prep day: _____
- [ ] 📖 Read "Make Healthy Foods a Delight."
- [ ] ✎ What healthy foods do you already delight in? _____
    _____
    _____
    _____
    _____

- [ ] ✎ What healthy foods do you want to delight in? _____
    _____
    _____
    _____
    _____

- [ ] 📖 Read "Make Time for Prayer and Meditation."

☐ ✎ Copy Isaiah 58:6. _____
_____
_____
_____

☐ ✎ What are your prayer goals for this time of fasting? _____
_____
_____
_____
_____

☐ 📖 Read "Make Praises."

☐ ✎ Copy Psalm 118: 24. _____
_____
_____
_____

☐ ✎ Start your list of praises: _____
_____
_____
_____
_____
_____
_____
_____

- [ ] ▶ Watch "Your Goals."
- [ ] ✎ Pray over and write your goals here:

_____
_____
_____
_____
_____
_____
_____

- [ ] ✎ Make your own grocery list (or use the one on pages 21 – 23 of the *Daniel Fast Book*).
- [ ] 📋 Consider getting a 3-ring binder or folder to keep all your Daniel Fast resources in (organization helps with intentionality!).
- [ ] ▶ Watch Bonus Video "Breakfast Ideas."

Notes/Highlights for group discussion session: _____

_____
_____
_____
_____
_____
_____

Questions to bring up in group discussion session: _____

_____
_____
_____
_____
_____
_____

Week 1

- ☐ 🗒️ Go grocery shopping!
- ☐ 🍲 Complete a week's worth of meal prep. Everything is here! The menu, the grocery list, and the recipes for week 1.

Daniel Fast Week 1 Sample Menu

	Mon	Tues	Wed	Thu	Fri	Sat	Sun
Breakfast	Muesli Mix Almond Milk & Banana	DF Smoothie Toast w/ Nut Butter	Overnight Oatmeal w/Fruit	DF Smoothie Toast w/ Nut Butter	Muesli Mix Almond Milk & Banana	Toast w/ Nut Butter Apple	Overnight Oatmeal w/Fruit
Snack	Bean Hummus Carrots & Broccoli	Krunch Kale Krisps	Dried Fruit Balls	Krunch Kale Krisps	Bean Hummus Carrots & Broccoli	Dried Fruit Balls	Krunch Kale Krisps
Lunch	Rice w/Steamed Veggies	Vegetarian Chili Carrot & Celery Sticks	Lentil Salad Orange	Rice w/Steamed Veggies	Healthy Tuscan White Bean Salad Fruit Kabobs	Vegetarian Chili Carrot & Celery Sticks	Lentil Salad Orange
Dinner	Vegetarian Chili Green Salad w/Orange Slices	Nutty Veggie Burger w/Mango Salsa Broccoli	Italian Vegetable Soup Turkish Salad & Chips	3-Bean Indian Dal w/Green Salad Israelite Unleavened Bread w/oil	Nutty Veggie Burger w/Mango Salsa Broccoli	3-Bean Indian Dal w/Green Salad Israelite Unleavened Bread w/oil	Italian Vegetable Soup Turkish Salad

Daniel Fast Week 1 Custom Menu

	Mon	Tues	Wed	Thu	Fri	Sat	Sun
Breakfast							
Snack							
Lunch							
Dinner							

Daniel Fast Week 1 Sample Menu Grocery List

Produce
Apple
Baby Carrots
Baby Spinach
Banana
Blackberries
Blueberries
Broccoli
Butternut Squash
Cantaloupe
Carrots
Celery
Coconut Meat
Cucumber
Fresh Basil
Fresh Garlic
Fresh Mint
Fresh Parsley
Green Beans
Green Bell Pepper
Green Cabbage
Green Lettuce
Green Onions
Kale
Lemon Juice
Lime Juice
Mango
Mixed Greens
Mushrooms
Navel Orange
Pimento
Pineapple
Plum Tomatoes
Raspberries
Red Bell Pepper
Red Onion
Strawberries
Sweet Onion
Tomato
Zucchini

Pantry
Black Beans
Black Olives
Brown Rice
Cannellini Beans
Chickpeas
Cornmeal
Diced Tomatoes
Dried Apricots
Dried Unsweetened Cranberries
Lentils
Oats
Pitted Dates
Pitted Prunes
Protein Powder
Red Kidney Beans
Raisins
Sunflower Seed Butter
Unsweetened Coconut Flakes
Vegetable Broth
Whole Grain Bread
Whole Wheat Flour

Seeds & Nuts
Cashews
Chia
Flax
Hemp
Pecans
Sesame Seeds
Sunflower Seeds
Walnuts

Oil & Spices
Apple Cider Vinegar
Avocado Oil
Balsamic Vinegar
Black Pepper
Cayenne Pepper
Celery Seed
Chia Seeds
Chili Powder
Cilantro
Cinnamon
Coconut Oil
Coriander
Cumin
Extra Virgin Olive Oil
Garlic Powder
Ground Ginger
Italian Seasoning
Oregano
Red Wine Vinegar
Sage
Sea Salt
Tahini
Tomato Sauce
White Pepper
White Wine Vinegar

Cold & Frozen
Frozen Blueberries
Orange Juice
Pineapple Juice
Unsweetened Almond Milk

🌿 Day 1 - Seek the Strength from the Holy Spirit

Whether this is the first time fasting or the beginning of another fast, it all begins with the first day. We have chosen the Daniel Fast in a desire to draw closer to God through fasting. "This is the day the Lord has made. Let us rejoice and be glad in it."

We can be glad because He is going to help us with whatever comes our way today. We can be confident because nothing is too hard for the Lord Jesus!

You have prayed about fasting. It is important to ask for strength during the fast. The Holy Spirit is within us, and we can depend on Him as our body responds to the fasting process.

When our stomachs growl today, we can rest and abide by the grace and truth that He is there helping us get through these challenges. Set aside some time during the usual mealtime to pray and meditate on a favorite Scripture passage. It is good to start a journal. Be sure to drink plenty of water so that the toxins and waste can be easily flushed from your system.

Revelation - Bible verse(s): _____

_____

_____

Inspiration - What is God speaking to your heart? _____

_____

_____

Illumination - Moving into action/God working through you: _____

_____

_____

Praises: _____

_____

_____

_____

☐ ▶ Watch "Daniel Fast Meal Prepping with Rhonda". Gather ingredients for Muesli, Hummus, and Salad to make the recipe along with Rhonda.

Day 2 - The Beauty of Fasting

The stomach has a capacity that is just waiting to be filled. That's why you're experiencing such hunger. God has built into your body an automatic response. When your "tank is empty," you want to fill it. Because of that mechanism, we get in the habit of thinking often about food.

Morning, mid-morning, noon, mid-afternoon, evening and even late evening, we go looking for things to satisfy our appetite. Yet during this fast, our focus is to be in a different capacity. We are to hunger for a deeper relationship with our loving Lord. After all, our fellowship with God is even more satisfying than food. So, each time you sense that hunger, turn your mind to spiritual things.

Recognize your need for God's love, mercy, wisdom, and strength. Just think how wonderful it will be to concentrate, those five or six times a day, on God instead of food! That is the beauty of fasting.

Revelation - Bible verse(s): _____

_____

_____

_____

Inspiration - What is God speaking to your heart? _____

_____

_____

Illumination - Moving into action/God working through you: _____

_____

_____

Praises: _____

_____

_____

_____

☐ 📱 Read "Daniel Fast Menu and Recipes - Week 1."

🌿 Day 3 - Drink Plenty of Water

The marvels of fasting are working on your body. Cells and tissues are releasing those toxins that have built up in your system. This is a very healthy change for you. But if you're not careful, you'll feel the effects of those toxins as they wind their way towards elimination. For example, you could have a really severe headache or even some muscle tension.

Therefore, the best thing you can do is to drink plenty of water. That will help flush those toxins out of your body. Even if you don't feel thirsty, drink some more. While you're drinking lots of water and eliminating these poisons from your body, this is a good time to seek inner purity. Jesus said we are to thirst for righteousness. (Matt. 5:6)

During this fast, you may find improper personal attitudes and motivations coming to light. Let the Holy Spirit deal with those, just as if they were poison. You'll feel better!

Revelation - Bible verse(s): _____

_____

_____

_____

Inspiration - What is God speaking to your heart? _____

_____

_____

Illumination - Moving into action/God working through you: _____

_____

_____

Praises: _____

_____

_____

_____

☐ 📖 Read "Testimony: God is Already Revealing Himself."

☐ ✎ Copy John 6:26-27. _____
_____
_____
_____
_____
_____
_____
_____
_____
_____
_____
_____
_____

✿ Day 4 - Meditate on a Bible Verse

Did you know your body expects and depends on routine? As the day dawns, you desire nourishment. At midday, you seek more energy. At the close of the day, it's time to replenish your reserves. But on this day of fasting, let those signals turn your attention to a different nourishment: the Word of God.

Truths from the Bible actually feed your soul. They strengthen you, wiser and spiritually healthy. So each time you think of food today, divert your thoughts to Scripture. If you have your Bible nearby, read a significant section and ask God's Spirit to use it as divine nourishment.

If you can't have a Bible with you during the day, then select a verse or two that you can memorize and carry with you. During your normal mealtimes, meditate on those verses and let them nurture your spiritual vitality. Use your hunger as a tool to help you grow stronger with the Lord.

Revelation - Bible verse(s): _____
_____
_____
_____

Inspiration - What is God speaking to your heart? _____
_____
_____

Illumination - Moving into action/God working through you: _____
_____
_____

Praises: _____
_____
_____
_____
_____

☐ Read "What is a Name?"

☐ Copy the 4 names of God covered in this section and what they mean:
   1. _____
   2. _____
   3. _____
   4. _____

☐ Record your reflections on this section: _____
_____
_____
_____
_____
_____
_____
_____
_____
_____

❦ Day 5 - Focus on the Lord

Today will probably be a difficult one physically. Your stomach will ache for attention and your body will complain that it's not getting the treatment it craves. Yet this denial of self can be a wonderful thing. It throws into stark contrast the way your spirit has probably felt in the past.

Sometimes your spiritual life was not being fed, and you paid attention primarily to your physical desires. On this day, however, the tables are turned.

It's time for your Lord to be in the spotlight. He wants your focus to be more on Him and the quality of your relationship. It's all right if your flesh suffers a little today. It's worth the price if your walk with Jesus is prospering.

God hungers for you and desires a deep bond with you, one that goes beyond casual discipleship. He wants to be Number One in your life. As your body reminds you of its hunger, let that point you to God's passionate love for you.

Revelation - Bible verse(s): _____

_____

_____

_____

Inspiration - What is God speaking to your heart? _____

_____

_____

Illumination - Moving into action/God working through you: _____

_____

_____

Praises: _____

_____

_____

_____

☐ Read "What is Your Identity?"

☐ Read Daniel chapters 1 and 10.

Day 6 - Establish a Personal Rapport with God

It is fatiguing to fight against the desires of the flesh, isn't it? Food is pleasurable to the senses and your body is crying out for some gratification. This is a good time to remind yourself that this fast brings pleasure to the Lord, not your flesh.

As you place your physical desires to the side and concentrate on your love relationship with God, the Lord is pleased. He has wanted to draw nearer to you and this is the opportunity for you both to be closer together.

According to James 4:8, when we draw near to God, He actually moves closer to us spiritually. Are you ready for that kind of encounter with the Creator? Perhaps you've already sensed a renewed intimacy with the Lord. If so, take some time today to praise the Lord. What a privilege it is to have a personal rapport with the Almighty!

Revelation - Bible verse(s): _____

_____

_____

_____

Inspiration - What is God speaking to your heart? _____

_____

_____

Illumination - Moving into action/God working through you: _____

_____

_____

Praises: _____

_____

_____

_____

☐ 📖 Read "What About Your Friends."

☐ ✎ Write the 4 takeaways from Daniel listed in this section and any others that you may have.

1. _____
2. _____
3. _____
4. _____
5. _____
6. _____
7. _____

☐ ✎ List godly, faithful friends who encourage you, hold you accountable, and walk with you on your journey with God.

_____
_____
_____

☐ ✎ Copy one of the "Fear not" verses. Consider putting it on a note card for your purse or putting it as a weekly/bi-weekly reminder on your phone.

_____
_____
_____
_____

🌱 Day 7 - Cleanse on the Inside

Your body is adapting to the lack of food. Your stomach is shrinking, and your cells are shedding those toxins. But today, let's not think about what's happening with your body. Let's focus instead on your soul.

A fast can become a time of heightened spiritual awareness. During this experience, let God speak to you about pollutants from this world that have embedded themselves in your life. Are there attitudes, beliefs, or viewpoints that negatively affect your relationship with God and with others?

Getting rid of worldly filth can be even more challenging than fasting. Today, ask the Lord to search your heart and help you in identifying those things that need to change. Confess those sins to the Savior and let him cleanse your heart. He will wash away the impurities, leaving you free once again to walk in the truth. This encounter with God may not be easy, but you certainly don't want to avoid it. After this period of repentance, you'll feel so much better.

When you take a bath or shower today, praise the Lord that He is cleansing you inside and rejoice as water washes away dead skin cells and eliminates odors. It is great to feel "clean" before the Lord! Praise His Name!

Revelation - Bible verse(s): _____
_____
_____

Inspiration - What is God speaking to your heart? _____
_____
_____

Illumination - Moving into action/God working through you: _____
_____

Praises: _____
_____
_____

☐ ▶ Watch Bonus Video "Sweet Potato Salad Recipe."

☐ 📝 Go grocery shopping!

Notes/Highlights for group discussion session: _____
_____
_____
_____
_____
_____
_____
_____

Questions to bring up in group discussion session: _____
_____
_____
_____
_____
_____
_____
_____

Week 2

- ☐ Go grocery shopping (if you haven't already)!
- ☐ Complete a week's worth of meal prep.

Daniel Fast Week 2 Sample Menu

	Mon	Tues	Wed	Thu	Fri	Sat	Sun
Breakfast	Yummy Brown Rice with Apple	Quick & Easy Breakfast Bar Banana	Pancakes with Fruit Sauce	Fruitful Rice Pudding	Quick & Easy Breakfast Bar Banana	Fruitful Rice Pudding	Pancakes with Fruit Sauce
Snack	White Bean Dip Carrot & Celery Sticks	Frozen Grapes	Healthy Banana Cookies	White Bean Dip Carrot & Celery Sticks	Frozen Grapes	Healthy Banana Cookies	White Bean Dip Carrot & Celery Sticks
Lunch	Tuscan Villa Bean Soup Carrot Sticks	Butternut Squash Soup Tabouli (Stuffed in Tomatoes)	Steamed Vegetables with Quinoa	Vegetable Fried Rice Wrap	Tuscan Villa Bean Soup Carrot Sticks	Vegetable Fried Rice Wrap	Butternut Squash Soup Tabouli (Stuffed in Tomatoes)
Dinner	Veggie Medley Tomato Sauce w/Spaghetti Squash Oven Roasted Broccoli & Cauliflower	Moroccan Vegetable Stew Green Salad w/Vinaigrette	Hummus & Veggie Wrap Green Salad w/Orange Slices	Marinated Vegetable Salad Fresh Strawberries	Veggie Medley Tomato Sauce w/Spaghetti Squash Oven Roasted Broccoli & Cauliflower	Moroccan Vegetable Stew Green Salad w/Vinaigrette	Marinated Vegetable Salad Fresh Strawberries

Daniel Fast Week 2 Custom Menu

	Mon	Tues	Wed	Thu	Fri	Sat	Sun
Breakfast							
Snack							
Lunch							
Dinner							

Daniel Fast Week 2 Menu Grocery List

Produce

Apple
Asparagus
Avocado
Banana
Blueberries
Broccoli
Butternut Squash
Carrots
Cauliflower
Celery
Cherry Tomatoes
Cucumber
Fresh Basil
Fresh Dill
Fresh Garlic
Fresh Mint
Fresh Oregano
Grapes
Green Bell Pepper
Green Lettuce
Green Onion
Lemon Juice
Mixed Greens
Mushrooms
Navel Orange
Parsley
Raspberries
Red Onion
Red Bell Pepper
Red Potato
Roma Tomato
Romaine
Rosemary
Rutabaga
Scallions
Spaghetti Squash
Strawberries
Summer Squash
Sweet Onion
Sweet Potato
Tomato
Turnip
Zucchini

Pantry

Baking Powder
Baking Soda
Brown Rice
Bulgur Wheat
Cannellini Beans
Chickpeas
Chocolate Protein Powder
Crushed Pineapple
Dried Unsweetened Cranberries
Kamut Flour
Organic Ketchup
Pearl Barley
Quinoa
Raisins
Rolled Oats
Stevia
Tomato Paste
Unsweetened Applesauce
Vegetable Broth
White Navy Beans
Whole Wheat Tortilla
Whole Wheat Flour

Seeds & Nuts

Cashews

Oil & Spices

Allspice
Almond Extract
Apple Cider Vinegar
Balsamic Vinegar
Bay Leaf
Black Pepper
Bragg's Liquid Aminos
Cayenne Pepper
Cinnamon
Coconut Oil
Coriander
Cumin
Dried Rosemary
Dry Mustard
Extra Virgin Olive Oil
Garlic Powder
Ground Ginger
Nutmeg
Oregano
Red Pepper Flakes
Red Wine Vinegar
Rice Vinegar
Safflower Oil
Sea Salt
Thyme
Toasted Sesame Oil
Vanilla Extract
Whole Cloves

Cold & Frozen

Hummus
Orange Juice

Day 8 - Turn Mealtimes into Moments of Prayer

For many of us, food has been a stronghold. It has exerted power over us. We would schedule our days around eating, turn to snacks for comfort, and even hide from the pressures of the world inside our fortress of food. But no more! The walls of that stronghold are crumbling around us.

We are now free!

Doesn't it feel wonderful to know that food is not your master?

As you experience freedom, this is a prime opportunity to think about your friends and family who may be imprisoned by other strongholds. Food is not the only prison that we can build. Our loved ones may be dominated by drugs, alcohol, pornography, IPhones, clothes, possessions, etc. What can you do about it?

Turn your mealtimes today into moments of intercession. Take your mind off yourself and pray for those who are unknowingly in bondage. Ask the Lord to help them become free, just as He's helped you during this fast.

Revelation - Bible verse(s): _____

_____

_____

Inspiration - What is God speaking to your heart? _____

_____

_____

Illumination - Moving into action/God working through you: _____

_____

_____

Praises: _____

_____

_____

_____

☐ ▶ Watch "Daniel Fast Meal Prepping with Rhonda" Gather ingredients for the Daniel Fast Smoothie and Vegetable Fried Rice Wrap to make the recipe along with Rhonda.

🌿 Day 9 - Remember This: You are Never Alone

During a fast, we become painfully aware of our weaknesses. Yes, we have hunger pangs and other aches that remind us of our mortal condition. But even more, we see how weak we are inwardly.

Our strength of will is challenged and we feel that we may fail in our resolve to fast. Our feelings are no longer dampened by the pleasures of food, and we are shocked by some of our reactions to life. The only bright hope in all this is the Lord. When we are weak, He is strong.

God never expects you to achieve life's goals on your own. He designed you to need Him.

That's why He's provided promises for you and me. He has opened an account in your name and it's full of strength, wisdom, perseverance, joy, peace and love. All we have to do is access it through faith. This email is a gentle reminder to you that you're not alone in this journey. The Lord's promises are only a breath away.

Revelation - Bible verse(s): _____
_____
_____

Inspiration - What is God speaking to your heart? _____
_____
_____

Illumination - Moving into action/God working through you: _____
_____
_____

Praises: _____
_____
_____
_____

☐ ▶ Watch "Don't Quit."

Day 10 - Yes, You Can Do it!

Friends and family may tell you that this fast makes little sense. You may have even had such thoughts from time to time. But fasting is not a normal experience. It is a planned opportunity to "Trust in the LORD with all your heart, and lean not on your own understanding" (Prov. 3:5).

This far into the fast, you are probably being tempted to revert back to your old eating patterns. You hear the voices of caring friends telling you to put an end to this practice. Or you "hear your body", telling you to cease fasting and get back to normal life. Actually, you find yourself at a crossroads. Will you listen to others, or will you trust in the Lord and His strength? Will you yield to your body or to the encouraging whispers of the Holy Spirit?

Let me cheer you on today: don't give up! Listen to the Lord, not to the world nor to the flesh. God will give you the support and perseverance that you need. You can do it!

Revelation - Bible verse(s): _____

_____

_____

Inspiration - What is God speaking to your heart? _____

_____

_____

Illumination - Moving into action/God working through you: _____

_____

_____

Praises: _____

_____

_____

_____

☐ Read "The Benefits of Detoxing Our Body."

Day 11 - Share God's Love with Others

During these days of fasting, God has undoubtedly been teaching you things about yourself and about Himself. It's because of your physical discomforts that you've realized your deepest desires and attitudes.

Whereas those things remained hidden while your flesh was being satisfied, they've now been revealed and brought into the light. You've talked with the Lord and have attained a new depth of relationship. Isn't that exciting?

Perhaps today you'll want to discuss those issues even further with Him.

While it's encouraging to receive fresh insights, they're not intended for you alone. It's good to share the truth with those you love, with those who need to hear about God's love and faithfulness. You may know someone close to you who is discouraged and can't see the light of God. They're going through a dark time. Why not share with them what God has shown you? It could make a difference in their lives.

Revelation - Bible verse(s): _____
_____
_____
_____

Inspiration - What is God speaking to your heart? _____
_____
_____

Illumination - Moving into action/God working through you: _____
_____
_____

Praises: _____
_____
_____
_____

☐ Read "Testimony: Daniel Fast Success Story."

Day 12 - Write a Letter to God

As you continue down this pathway of fasting, you'll find that it's truly a sweet journey. You're experiencing victory and an extra measure of health. It is important, however, to lay down some markers along the road.

Someday you'll want to return to those markers and recall the successes you've had with God. There are a couple of ways to do this. The first is to choose good Bible verses you can associate with this time of fasting and triumph.

Memorize them today and then meditate on them in the last half of your commitment.

You may also want to write a letter to God, expressing your appreciation for His strength and wisdom during this difficult time. You can mention to Him all that you've learned and the ways you've grown. Tuck that letter away in your Bible or in your bedside table. Later, you'll enjoy reflecting on all that God has done for you.

Revelation - Bible verse(s): _____

_____

_____

_____

Inspiration - What is God speaking to your heart? _____

_____

_____

Illumination - Moving into action/God working through you: _____

_____

_____

Praises: _____

_____

_____

_____

☐ ✍ Write your letter to God.

Day 13 - Acknowledge Your Accomplishment

Some days of fasting are harder than others. It's kind of like running a race. Sometimes you feel you've gotten your "second wind" while other times you feel near fatigue. How are you doing today?

It's probably fairly difficult for you to keep going at this point. And that's precisely when you need to turn your gaze away from yourself and towards Jesus.

Look today at Hebrews 12:1-2. Jesus endured physical pains that we can hardly imagine. He may have been tempted to give up, to stop his commitment to die on the cross. But Jesus didn't quit. He looked forward to the end goal. He knew that joy and victory were just across the finish line.

Won't you do the same today? Look ahead to the worthy accomplishment you'll have made. Contemplate the thrill of being victorious.

Then ask the Father to help you persevere, in the same way He helped Jesus remain on the cross. This can literally be a life-changing experience.

Revelation - Bible verse(s): _____

_____

_____

Inspiration - What is God speaking to your heart? _____

_____

_____

Illumination - Moving into action/God working through you: _____

_____

_____

Praises: _____

_____

_____

_____

☐ ✎ What are your thoughts/reflections at this point in the fast?

_____

_____

_____

_____

Day 14 - Count Your Treasures

As you complete this second week of fasting, take the time to complete an inventory. No, don't list everything you wish you could have eaten. It's time to jot down the values and priorities that you've seen hiding deep in your heart. What things have revealed themselves as being important to you?

After noting your top ten treasures, turn your attention to the Lord. What would you say are His top ten priorities? Does your list align with His?

This is one of the greatest challenges to a child of God: submitting our cherished values to Him. As we do this, our number one passion in life will be to glorify God. Isn't that actually why you're committed to this fast? You want the Lord to be glorified through your body, mind, and spirit.

Therefore, ask the Holy Spirit today to fill you, to control you, so that all you do will be for the glory of God.

Revelation - Bible verse(s): _____
_____
_____
_____

Inspiration - What is God speaking to your heart? _____
_____
_____

Illumination - Moving into action/God working through you: _____
_____
_____

Praises: _____
_____
_____
_____
_____

☐ ▶ Watch Bonus Video "Brown Rice with Apples Recipe."

☐ 📋 Go grocery shopping!

Notes/Highlights for group discussion session: _____

_____

_____

_____

_____

_____

_____

Questions to bring up in group discussion session: _____

_____

_____

_____

_____

_____

_____

Week 3

☐ 🗒 Go grocery shopping! (If you haven't already)

☐ 🍲 Complete a week's worth of meal prep.

Daniel Fast Week 3 Sample Menu

	Mon	Tues	Wed	Thu	Fri	Sat	Sun
Breakfast	Cream of Wheat with Almond Milk and Applesauce	DF Breakfast Burrito	Very Berry Drink Toast with Peanut Butter	Cream of Wheat with Almond Milk and Applesauce	DF Cherry Berry Muesli	Very Berry Drink Toast with Peanut Butter	DF Breakfast Burrito
Snack	Fruit Plate Almonds	Krunch Kale Crisps	Crispy Beans Fruit Slices	Hummus with Veggies	Healthy Banana Cookies	Fruit Plate Almonds	Krunch Kale Crisps
Lunch	Tex Mex Chili Green Salad with Orange Slices	Lentil Soup Celery with Peanut Butter	Chickpea Salad Spelt Chapatti	Tex Mex Chili Green Salad with Orange Slices	Lentil Soup Celery with Peanut Butter	Savory Stuffed Peppers Carrot & Celery Sticks	Chickpea Salad Spelt Chapatti
Dinner	Sweet Potato Pie Mideast Pilaf	Popeye Burgers Fruit Plate	Spanish Paella Green Salad with Vinaigrette	Italian Vegetable Soup Green Salad with Corn Chips	Turkish Salad Vegetable Soup	Spanish Paella Green Salad with Vinaigrette	Popeye Burgers Fruit Plate

Daniel Fast Week 3 Custom Menu

	Mon	Tues	Wed	Thu	Fri	Sat	Sun
Breakfast							
Snack							
Lunch							
Dinner							

Daniel Fast Week 3 Sample Menu Grocery List

Produce

- Avocado
- Baby Carrots
- Baby Spinach
- Banana
- Bell Peppers
- Blackberries
- Blueberries
- Broccoli
- Carrot
- Cauliflower
- Celery
- Collard Greens
- Corn
- Cucumber
- Eggplant
- Fresh Garlic
- Fresh Mint
- Fresh Oregano
- Fresh Parsley
- Grapes
- Green Apple
- Green Beans
- Green Cabbage
- Green Lettuce
- Green Onion
- Honeydew Melon
- Jalapeno Pepper
- Kale
- Kiwi
- Lemon Juice
- Lime Juice
- Mixed Greens
- Mushrooms
- Navel Orange
- Radishes
- Raspberries
- Red Onion
- Russet Potato
- Strawberries
- Sweet Onion
- Sweet Potato
- Tomato
- Yellow Onion
- Yellow Potato

Pantry

- Basmati Rice
- Black Beans
- Black Olives
- Brown Rice
- Brown Rice Tortilla
- Bulgur Wheat
- Cashew Butter
- Chickpeas
- Chocolate Protein Powder
- Corn Meal
- Dark Chocolate Powder
- Diced Tomatoes
- Dried Apricots
- Dried Unsweetened Cranberries
- Lentils
- Peanut Butter
- Pearl Barley
- Raisins
- Red Kidney Beans
- Rolled Oats
- Salsa
- Spelt Flour
- Steel Cut Oats
- Stevia
- Stewed Tomatoes
- Tahini
- Tomato Paste
- Tomato Sauce
- Unsweetened Applesauce
- Unsweetened Shredded Coconut
- Vegetable Broth
- White Kidney Beans
- Whole Grain Bread
- Whole Wheat Matzo

Seeds & Nuts

- Almonds
- Cashews
- Flax Seed
- Pecans

Oils & Spices

- Apple Cider Vinegar
- Balsamic Vinegar
- Basil
- Bay Leaf
- Black Pepper
- Bragg's Liquid Aminos
- Cardamom
- Cayenne Pepper
- Chili Powder
- Cilantro
- Cinnamon
- Cloves
- Coriander
- Cumin
- Dijon Mustard
- Dried Onion Flakes
- Extra Virgin Olive Oil
- Garlic Powder
- Italian Seasoning
- Oregano
- Paprika
- Parsley
- Red Pepper Flakes
- Rosemary
- Saffron
- Sea Salt
- Seasoned Salt
- Smoked Paprika
- Thyme
- Turmeric
- Vanilla Extract
- Wine Vinegar

Cold & Frozen

- Apple Juice
- Frozen Corn
- Frozen Green Beans
- Frozen Spinach
- Pomegranate Juice
- Unsweetened Almond Milk
- Unsweetened Coconut Yogurt

Day 15 - Listen for God's Words of Encouragement

Week Three! Praise the Lord! It's exciting that you have persevered, that God has helped you make it thus far. Whatever you do, don't stop drinking plenty of water. Keep yourself well hydrated. That's the key to staying healthy during this period of fasting.

Can you glance into the distance, towards the end of this week? There is a finish line, and it's already coming into view. Don't think of it as being far away. In fact, see yourself as actually completing the fast.

View the moment, by faith, when you cross the goal and seal your victory. Consider it today to be a "done deal." You will make it. Gaze on that coming success, knowing that you'll get there by walking in the Spirit, not in the flesh.

As you enter this final chapter of your journey, ask the Lord to reveal Himself in a fresh way. Keep listening for his gentle whispers of encouragement.

Revelation - Bible verse(s): _____
_____
_____
_____

Inspiration - What is God speaking to your heart? _____
_____
_____

Illumination - Moving into action/God working through you: _____
_____
_____

Praises: _____
_____
_____
_____

☐ ▶ Watch "Daniel Fast Meal Prepping with Rhonda." (Gather ingredients for the Healthy Banana Cookie and Black Bean Soup to make the recipes along with Rhonda.)

Day 16 - Show and Express Your Praises

Would you say that these past two weeks have been a time of sacrifice? Absolutely! In fact, you have been a living sacrifice, just as Paul mentioned in Romans 12:1-2. Pause for a moment and read this passage anew.

Remind yourself of what you have been experiencing. You have presented your body to the Lord in order to make it more pure and acceptable to Him. This has been a time of genuine worship.

Also, you have undergone a transformation of your mind. You've discovered a fresh hunger for God and new desires for spiritual health.

As you move forward in this final week of fasting, let this be a time of celebration. You have much for which to be thankful. God has proven His faithfulness to you. And you are enjoying a new level of health, not just outwardly but inwardly.

Let your praise show! May others see that you're walking in victory because of your mighty Lord.

Revelation - Bible verse(s): _____
_____
_____

Inspiration - What is God speaking to your heart? _____
_____
_____

Illumination - Moving into action/God working through you: _____
_____
_____

Praises: _____
_____
_____
_____

☐ ▶ Watch "Finish Strong."

Day 17 - Create a Plan

This fast has probably been unlike anything you've ever experienced. You've battled with your own flesh, wrestled with your feelings and altered your daily habits. Has anything taken you by surprise?

Perhaps you didn't know how much this would affect your inner life. Or you've discovered a new strength that you didn't think you had. In any case, you've had some wonderful, unanticipated revelations. You've discovered a new depth of truth.

One of the reasons you've had these experiences is because you've been spending more time with Jesus, the Truth. Hasn't it been magnificent? Instead of eating in your "normal routine," you've been making healthy choices, talking to and listening to the Spirit. But what will you do once the fast is completed? Will you continue to have those precious moments with the Lord?

Now is the time to start planning how you will carve out moments with God, once your life returns to its normal pace. This is a precious treasure that you don't want to lose.

Revelation - Bible verse(s): _____

_____

_____

Inspiration - What is God speaking to your heart? _____

_____

_____

Illumination - Moving into action/God working through you: _____

_____

_____

Praises: _____

_____

_____

_____

☐ Read "The Gift of Prayer."

🌿 Day 18 - Meditate on Love

Why have you been fasting? That may seem to be a silly question, now that you're so close to reaching your goal. But it's important to determine your motivation. Was it solely because you wanted to lose weight? Or were you primarily driven by the desire to detoxify your body and experience increased health?

I hope it's been more than that. The purest impulse for fasting can be found in 1 Corinthians 13:1-3. Love is the driving force that won't fall flat or take you down a dead end road. By fasting out of a deep love for God, you discover how crucial it is to have a solid relationship with the Lord.

Weight can fluctuate with time. It can't be your firm source of hope. And your health is not guaranteed. Things can change in a heartbeat. The only thing that you can count on is your Savior. Jesus said that he would never leave us or forsake us. In fact, he's with you today, ready to help you as you near the end of this fast. Praise the Lord!

Please meditate and "chew on" on 1 Corinthians 13 today. Spend time "loving on" the Lord today and receive His wonderful love with deeper appreciation in a fresh way.

Revelation - Bible verse(s): _____

_____

_____

Inspiration - What is God speaking to your heart? _____

_____

_____

Illumination - Moving into action/God working through you: _____

_____

_____

Praises: _____

_____

_____

_____

☐ 📖 Read "Testimony: Finished the Daniel Fast and Ready to Move on to More!"

☐ List the gifts of prayer (covered in the course and any others you've experienced)

_____ _____
_____ _____
_____ _____
_____ _____
_____ _____
_____ _____
_____ _____
_____ _____

Day 19 - Sing to the Lord

You have had to tell yourself "no" so many times during the past couple of weeks. Your body has repeatedly asked for food and you've had to stay firm in your resolve. But this fast hasn't been about rules, right?

Fasting is about freedom! It's about telling your body that it won't be your master. Yea! You aren't obligated to obey its impulses.

You have only one Master and that is Jesus. With that kind of freedom, there is joy. Do you feel that deep sense of peace and fulfillment today? You have issued a declaration of independence from your fleshly desires. The skirmishes have been frequent, yet you've come through them victoriously. Look up Galatians 5:1 and read it out loud.

Christ has made us free, free indeed! We are not slaves to our appetites any longer. Let us walk in this freedom and hold on to the truth with the strength of our beloved Master.

With that level of success, it's time to sing an anthem of freedom. You are stronger in your faith, purer in heart, and healthier in your body. Take the time today to actually celebrate and sing to the Lord. Make up a song that proclaims to God how much you appreciate your freedom in Christ. Sing your favorite praise songs in sweet worship to our King!

Revelation - Bible verse(s): _____
_____
_____

Inspiration - What is God speaking to your heart? _____
_____
_____

Illumination - Moving into action/God working through you: _____
_____
_____

Praises: _____
_____
_____
_____

☐ ▶ Watch Bonus Video "How to End the Daniel Fast"

☐ ✎ What benefits of the Daniel Fast are you taking into your everyday life?

_____

_____

_____

_____

_____

☐ ✎ Write out the 3 steps of ending the Daniel Fast without losing the benefits:
1. _____
2. _____
3. _____

Day 20 - Celebrate Your Freedom

Oh my! Tomorrow is the day! Are you getting really excited about completing the fast? It's going to be a day of glorious victory. So, what are you going to do about it? Treat it like a normal day? I hope not.

You need to have a special celebration, just like we do on Independence Day. You may not have any fireworks to shoot off, but you can do the next best thing. Prepare your spiritual sparklers!

Today is the time to plan your celebration event. Pick out all those favorite Bible verses that articulate what you want to say to God and to others. Have them lined out so you can give a litany of praise to the Lord.

Do you have some preferred praise songs? Get the words together and have them ready to use. It's time for you to celebrate your independence, your freedom. You have not been a slave to food during this fast. Rejoice!

Revelation - Bible verse(s): _____
_____
_____
_____

Inspiration - What is God speaking to your heart? _____
_____
_____

Illumination - Moving into action/God working through you: _____
_____
_____

Praises: _____
_____
_____
_____
_____

☐ ▶ Watch Finishing the Daniel Fast Coaching Call

Day 21 - Rejoice - You Made it!

You did it! Don't you feel like jumping up and down? This is truly an exciting moment. And yet I know what you're thinking. Even though you've been victorious, all you feel like doing is pointing to the Lord. He's the One who gives you strength each day. All praise goes to Him.

As you celebrate today, think back to all the obstacles you had to overcome. God gave you everything you needed to do the impossible. He supplied wisdom, encouragement and power. If it's at all possible, go for a walk today with God. With each step, count your multitude of blessings. God has been incredibly good to you during this season of fasting. Now go tell someone what the Lord has meant to you during this time of testing. Proclaim His goodness.

Please read Ephesians 3:16-21 and enjoy your victory lap! You've made it! Congratulations! The Lord is exalted and He is your eternal reward!

Revelation - Bible verse(s): _____
_____
_____
_____

Inspiration - What is God speaking to your heart? _____
_____
_____

Illumination - Moving into action/God working through you: _____
_____
_____

Praises: _____
_____
_____
_____

✎ Reflect on your Daniel Fast journey. What are your successes and praises?

_____
_____
_____
_____
_____
_____
_____
_____
_____
_____

✎ Write out your plan for ending the Daniel Fast for continuing with new, healthy eating habits. What are your physical, spiritual, and emotional health goals in the coming days and weeks?

_____
_____
_____
_____
_____
_____
_____
_____
_____
_____

Notes/Highlights for group discussion session: _____

_____
_____
_____
_____
_____
_____
_____

Questions to bring up in group discussion session: _____

_____
_____
_____
_____
_____
_____
_____

Recipes

Bean Hummus

Ingredients

1 ½ c cooked Chickpeas (substitute red, pinto, or black beans)
¼ c Tahini
2 T Lemon Juice
2 T Cilantro
⅛ t Cayenne Pepper
2 Green Onions
1 T Extra Virgin Olive Oil
1 clove Fresh Garlic
½ t Cumin or more as desired

Directions

1. Combine all ingredients in a food processor until smooth.
2. Season with salt and pepper to taste.
3. Serve with raw veggies of choice.

Best Hummus Ever Tip

If you want the creamiest hummus possible. Cook the beans, yes, cooked beans, in a pot with water and a teaspoon baking soda. Cook for 10 – 15 minutes until the skins come off. Then drain and add to recipe. You can also remove all the skins before adding to the recipe.

Your friends will wonder how you made the most delicious hummus ever!

Better Bean Burgers

Makes 5-6 Burgers – Great to Refrigerate or Freeze Leftovers!

Ingredients:

3 c cooked Kidney or Black Beans
1-2 cloves Fresh Garlic
3 T Tomato Paste
1 T Red Wine or Balsamic Vinegar
1 t Dijon mustard
¾ c Green Onions
¼ c Fresh Parsley

2 T Fresh Oregano
½ t Sea Salt
Black pepper to taste
1¼ c Rolled Oats
½ c Organic Corn
⅓ c Olives (optional)
¼ c Red Bell Pepper (optional)

Directions:

1. Chop the green onions, parsley, oregano, olives, and bell pepper. Chop/mince the garlic.
2. In a food processor or blender, combine the beans, garlic, tomato paste, vinegar, and mustard. Pulse until pureed.
3. Add the green onions, parsley, oregano, salt, and pepper to taste, and process to break up and blend.
4. Add the oats and pulse to begin to incorporate. Transfer the mixture to a large bowl and stir in the olives, corn and red pepper.
5. Refrigerate the mixture for 30-45 minutes.
6. Shape into patties with hands.
7. Cook the patties for 6 to 8 minutes per side, or until golden brown.

*Skillet Option: Lightly coat skillet with oil and cook on medium/ medium-high heat.
*Oven Option: Bake the patties for about 15-20 minutes at 400 ° on an oiled pan, flipping once through cooking. Delicious with salsa or guacamole.

Black Bean and Mango Salsa

Servings: 5-8

Ingredients:

1 c cooked Black Beans
2 Mangos
½ Red Pepper
½ Green Pepper
¾ c Pineapple Juice

½ c Lime Juice
½ c Fresh Cilantro
2 T Ground Cumin
1 sm. Jalapeno Pepper
Salt and Pepper to taste

Directions:

1. Peel, seed, and dice the mangos. Core, seed, and dice the bell peppers and jalapeno pepper. Chop the cilantro.
2. Combine all ingredients in a medium bowl. Adjust seasoning as desired.
3. Cover and refrigerate for at least 1 hour or up to 4 days.

Black Bean Dip

Ingredients

2 c Black Beans (cooked and cooled)
1 c Frozen Corn
2 stalks Green Onion
½ c Purple Onion
¼ c Cilantro

¾ c Grape Tomatoes
½ c Extra Virgin Olive Oil
3 T Cumin
3 Limes (Juiced)

Directions

1. Chop the green onion, purple onion, and grape tomatoes.
2. Drain the beans. Rinse the beans and corn in a colander.
3. Place all ingredients in a bowl, stir together, and chill for several hours.
4. Serve with chips, raw veggies, or on a salad.

Broccoli & Carrots

Ingredients

¼ t Sea Salt
2 Carrots
2 c Broccoli Florets

Directions

1. Bring a pot of water to boil and add the salt.
2. Add the carrots and cook for 5 minutes.
3. Add broccoli and continue cooking until the vegetables are tender.
4. Drain and serve.

Butternut Squash Soup

Ingredients

2 t Extra Virgin Olive Oil
1 Sweet Onion, peeled and chopped
3 cloves Fresh Garlic, crushed
2 t Cumin
3 c Butternut Squash, peeled and cubed
2 Sweet Potato, cut into chunks
1 Rutabaga, cut into chunks
1 Turnip, cut into chunks
4 c Vegetable Broth
1 ½ t Sea Salt
¼ Ground Black Pepper
1 Red Bell Pepper (optional)

Directions

1. Heat the oil in a large pot. Add the onion and sauté over medium heat until translucent.
2. Add the garlic and sauté until soft, but not brown.
3. Stir in the cumin and cook for 2-3 minutes.
4. Add the squash, sweet potato, rutabaga, and turnip. Stir to coat each piece with the onion/garlic mixture.
5. Add the vegetable broth and bring to a boil. Turn down the heat and simmer for 30-40 minutes.
6. Puree the mixture and thin the soup, if desired, with more broth.
7. Add salt, ground black pepper, and red pepper to taste.
8. Garnish with chopped parsley, cilantro, toasted pecans, and/or sunflower seeds.

When not following the Daniel Fast, this soup taste even better with some maple syrup.

Chickpea Salad

Ingredients

2 c cooked Chickpeas
2 Tomatoes
1 Cucumber
½ Red Onion
1 T Extra Virgin Olive Oil
2 T Lemon Juice
¼ t Sea Salt

Directions

1. Dice the tomato. Peel and chop the cucumber. Chop the onion.
2. Combine all the ingredients.

Classic Carrot Soup

Ingredients
4 c Carrots
2 T Extra Virgin Olive Oil
1 t Sea Salt
¼ t Ground Black Pepper
4 c Water
2 T Basil Leaves

Directions
1. Preheat oven to 425°.
2. Line a large baking sheet with foil or parchment paper.
3. Peel the carrots and cut them into ½ inch chunks.
4. Drizzle carrots with olive oil.
5. Spread carrots in a single layer on prepared baking sheet and roast for 25-30 minutes, stirring occasionally.
6. Move carrots to a medium saucepan and add water, salt, and pepper. Bring to boil, reduce heat and simmer for 5 minutes.
7. Chop basil.
8. Remove from heat and blend well with immersion blender until completely smooth. Garnish with basil.

Cream of Wheat with Almond Milk and Applesauce

Ingredients
1 c Water
2 T Unsweetened Almond Milk
¼ t Stevia
2 T Raisins
2 T Unsweetened Shredded Coconut
½ t Cinnamon
½ c Bulgur Wheat
½ t Vanilla Extract
¼ c Unsweetened Applesauce

Directions
1. Bring water to a boil.
2. Add all ingredients one at a time, adding the bulgur last.
3. Cover and simmer for 20 minutes.

Crispy Beans

Ingredients

1 c cooked White Kidney Beans; sub Red Kidney Beans

1 ½ t Extra Virgin Olive Oil

⅛ t Sea Salt

⅛ t Ground Black Pepper

1 ½ t Rosemary

Directions

1. Preheat the oven to 450°.
2. Rinse the beans and spread them on a baking sheet. Pat them dry.
3. Drizzle olive oil over the beans and stir until lightly coated.
4. Season with salt, pepper, and rosemary. (Feel free to add other spices.) Mix until well-coated.
5. Bake for 25-30 minutes, until brown and crispy.

Cumin Roasted Walnuts

Serving Size: 16

Ingredients:

2 c Walnuts

6 cloves Garlic

2 T Olive Oil

2 T ground Cumin

1 T Cumin Seed

1 t Sea Salt

2 T Honey

Directions:

1. Preheat the oven to 325°.
2. Chop the walnuts. Chop/mince the garlic.
3. Coarsely toast walnuts for 8-10 minutes.
4. Heat the oil in a medium skillet. Sauté the garlic until golden. Stir in ground cumin, cumin seed, salt, and honey.
5. Raise oven temperature to 375°.
6. Add toasted walnuts to skillet. Stir well to coat.
7. Spread evenly on a baking sheet and bake for 20 minutes or until golden. Cool thoroughly.

Daniel Fast Black Bean Soup
A favorite for years to come!

Ingredients
1 c Salsa
3 c cooked Black Beans
2 c Vegetable Broth
¼ c Unsweetened Coconut Yogurt, for topping
1 ½ t Chives, for topping

Directions
1. Heat the salsa in a large saucepan over medium heat, stirring constantly, for 5 minutes.
2. Stir in the beans and broth and heat to boiling. Reduce heat to low, cover, and simmer for 15 minutes.
3. Cool slightly.
4. Spoon ½ of the soup into a food processor or use an immersion blender and puree. Return pureed soup to the saucepan and heat through.
5. Serve with a dollop of coconut yogurt and chopped chives.

Daniel Fast Breakfast Burrito

Ingredients
½ Red Bell Pepper
3 Green Onions
2 Garlic Cloves
⅓ c Water
2 c cooked Black Beans
1 ½ t Bragg's Liquid Aminos
½ Tomato
5 oz Fresh Baby Spinach
⅓ c Ground Flaxseed
6 Brown Rice Tortillas

Directions
1. Chop bell pepper, green onion, and tomato. Chop/mince garlic.
2. Heat a large skillet and sauté peppers, onion, and garlic in water for 5 minutes.
3. Add the beans and liquid aminos, cooking another 5 minutes.
4. Remove from heat and mix in the tomatoes, desired seasoning or salt and pepper, spinach, and ground flaxseed.
5. Toast tortillas to soften and then add mixture and roll.

Daniel Fast Cabbage Rolls

Ingredients

12 Large Cabbage Leaves (regular or Napa)
2 T Olive Oil
1 c Chopped Onion
1 c Chopped Green Bell Pepper
2 cloves Garlic
8 oz Mushrooms (sliced)
½ t Sea Salt
¼ t Pepper
1 c Cooked Brown Rice

Directions

1. Preheat oven to 350 °.
2. Bring a large pot of water to boil; cook cabbage leaves, a few at a time for about 2 minutes or until softened. Drain and cool.
3. Heat oil over medium heat in a large skillet; sauté mushrooms, onion, bell pepper, and garlic until tender.
4. Add rice, salt, and pepper; stir gently until well blended.
5. Prepare a shallow 2-quart baking dish by brushing with vegetable oil.
6. Spoon mixture onto individual cabbage leaves; roll up and place seam-side down on baking dish.
7. Cover with foil and bake at 350 ° for 30 minutes.

Daniel Fast Berry Muesli

Ingredients

½ c Oats
½ c Pomegranate Juice
1 Banana
1 c Blueberries
1 Green Apple
2 T Ground Flaxseed
¼ c Unsweetened Almond Milk
3 T Unsweetened Coconut Yogurt
2 T Pecans

Directions

In the evening:

1. Soak the oats in the pomegranate juice. Let sit overnight.

In the morning:

2. Dice the banana, apple, and pecans.
3. Add all ingredients to the soaked oatmeal and mix well.

Daniel Fast Smoothie

Ingredients

1 c Water
⅔ c Strawberries
½ Banana
⅓ c Frozen Blueberries
1 c Baby Spinach
1 t Chia Seeds
1 T Flax or Hemp seeds (optional)
2 T Protein Powder (optional)

Directions

Put all ingredients in the blender, blend on high for 60 seconds, and enjoy. Add ice if desired for thickness and colder temperature.

Daniel Fast Sweet Potato Salad

Ingredients

6 Sweet Potatoes
1 Green Bell Pepper
½ Sweet Onion
1 ½ t Sea Salt
¼ Ground Black Pepper
1 ½ c Unsweetened Coconut Yogurt

Directions

1. Peel and chop the sweet potatoes. Chop the bell pepper and onion (finely).
2. In a large bowl, combine the sweet potatoes, pepper, onion, salt, and pepper.
3. Add a dash of pepper to the yogurt and stir in with the already combined ingredients.
4. Cover and refrigerate for at least 1 hour before serving.

Dried Fruit Balls

Ingredients

½ c Dried Apricots
¼ c Raisins
¼ c Pitted Prunes
¼ c Pitted Dates
½ c Pecans (or walnuts)
¼ c Unsweetened Coconut Flakes
¼ t Orange Zest
2 T Orange Juice

Directions

1. Grind the dried fruits together in a food processor.
2. Add the coconut, orange peel, orange juice, and half the nuts. Blend well.
3. Form the dough into balls. Roll in the remaining nuts.

Fall Harvest Salad

Ingredients

4 Stalks Green Onion
¼ c Extra Virgin Olive Oil
2 t Lemon Juice
2 t Bragg's Liquid Aminos
½ t Sea Salt
½ head Green Cabbage

1 Sweet Potato
½ Turnip
½ Dried Coconut
½ c Raisins
¼ c Almonds

Directions

1. Dice the onions. Shred the cabbage, sweet potato, and turnip.
2. Mix the onions, olive oil, lemon juice, liquid aminos, and salt. Stir thoroughly and refrigerate until ready to add to salad.
3. Combine the cabbage, sweet potato, turnip, coconut, raisins, and almonds. Add dressing.

Fast Italian Tomato-Bean Soup

Servings: 10

Recipe from The Antioxidant Diet; Robin Jeep and Dr. Couey

Ingredients:

4 c Organic Tomato Soup
   or Roasted Red Pepper Soup
4 c Frozen Spinach
4 c Broccoli
1 c Onion
2 c Frozen Peas or Green Beans

2 c Diced Tomatoes
3 c Carrot Juice
2 cloves Fresh Garlic
2 t Italian Seasoning
2-3 c cooked Red Kidney Beans
4 T Pine Nuts or Walnuts

Directions

1. Chop the broccoli, onion, and tomatoes. Chop/mince the garlic.
2. In a large pot, combine all ingredients except beans and nuts and simmer for 40 minutes.
3. Add beans and simmer for 10 additional minutes.
4. Serve topped with nuts.

Fruit Kabobs
Ingredients

¼ c Strawberries
¼ Pineapple
¼ c Blackberries
⅛ Cantaloupe

¼ c Blueberries
¼ c Raspberries
4 Barbeque Skewers

Directions
1. Wash the fruit.
2. Halve the strawberries; peel and cut the pineapple and cantaloupe into cubes.
3. Fill the skewers with one piece of fruit at a time, alternating the types of fruit.

Fruit Plate
Ingredients

1 ½ c Grapes
½ Honeydew Melon
⅔ c Blueberries

2 c Strawberries
1 Banana

Directions
Wash and slice fruit as desired. Feel free to mix and match with in-season fruit.

Fruitful Rice Pudding
Ingredients

1 c cooked Brown Rice
½ c Crushed Pineapple
2 T Raisins
⅓ c Hot Water

½ Banana
2 T Orange Juice
½ t Vanilla Extract
¼ t Almond Extract

Directions
1. Preheat the oven to 350°.
2. Mix the rice, pineapple, and raisins in an 8 x 8 casserole dish.
3. Process the remaining ingredients in a blender until smooth. Pour over the rice and fruit.
4. Bake for 45 minutes and serve hot.
5. Garnish with peach or banana slices.

Green Salad with Corn Chips

Ingredients

2 T Cornmeal

⅓ t Extra Virgin Olive Oil

1/16 t Sea Salt

1 ½ T Boiling Water

¼ c Mixed Greens

1 ⅛ t Red Wine Vinegar

Directions

1. Mix the cornmeal, olive oil, salt, and boiling water. Add more water if the dough feels too dry or crumbly.
2. Grease a flat baking pan or stone.
3. Roll out the dough very thin, with a cornmeal flour covered rolling pin to avoid sticking and bake at 400° for 8 minutes.
Salad
4. Wash and chop mixed greens and toss with red wine vinegar.
5. Remove chips from pan, flip chips, and bake 2 more minutes.
6. Serve salad with chips. Store the extra chips in an airtight container.

Green Salad with Orange Slices

Ingredients

2 c Mixed Greens

2 Naval Orange

¼ c Dried Unsweetened Cranberries

¼ c Apple Cider Vinegar

¼ c Balsamic Vinegar

¼ c Cashews

Directions

1. Wash and chop the greens.
2. Zest the orange over the greens.
3. Peel and pull apart the orange slices and add to the greens.
4. Add the dried cranberries, cashews, apple cider vinegar, and balsamic vinegar.

Healthy Banana Cookies
Too good to be called healthy

Ingredients
3 Bananas, ripe
1 c Raisins, or substitute chopped apples
2 c Rolled Oats
⅓ c Extra Virgin Olive Oil, or substitute applesauce
1 t Vanilla Extract

Directions
1. Preheat oven to 350°.
2. Mash the banana in a large bowl.
3. Stir in the oats, raisins, oil, and vanilla. Mix well and let mixture sit for 15 minutes.
4. Drop by teaspoons onto an ungreased cookie sheet.
5. Bake for 15-20 minutes.

Healthy Tuscan White Bean Salad

Ingredients
2 c cooked White Beans
1 clove Fresh Garlic
½ c Fresh Plum Tomatoes
¼ c Red Onion
¼ c fresh Italian Parsley
¼ c fresh Sage
2 T Extra Virgin Olive Oil
2 T Red Wine Vinegar
1 T Balsamic Vinegar
3 c Fresh Baby Spinach
Salt & Pepper

Directions
1. Chop/mince garlic.
2. Dice tomatoes, red onion, parsley, and sage.
3. In a medium bowl, combine white beans, garlic, tomatoes, red onion, parsley, and sage.
4. Combine vinegars and olive oil. Oil/vinegar over salad and toss.
5. Season with salt and pepper.
6. Spoon onto a bed of spinach. May be served at room temperature or chilled.

Hot and Spicy Hummus

Yield: 4 cups

Ingredients:

3 c cooked Garbanzo Beans, also known as Chickpeas
1 c Tahini
¼ c Lemon Juice
3 cloves Fresh Garlic
½ t White Pepper

1 t Sea Salt
1 t Ground Cumin
½ t Red Pepper Flakes
½ t Cayenne Pepper
½ t Black Pepper
¼ c Jalapeno Peppers

Directions:

1. Chop/mince the garlic. Finely dice the jalapeno pepper.
2. Puree garbanzo beans, tahini, and lemon juice until smooth, adding water as needed to make a creamy mixture.
2. Pour into a medium bowl and add remaining ingredients and stir well.
4. Chill to allow flavors to blend.

* Serving Ideas: Serve as a dip with raw veggies or add to a tossed salad as a dressing.
* This hummus is great in a whole grain wrap with lettuce, tomato and bean sprouts.
* The red pepper flakes, cayenne and jalapenos can be omitted or cut in half if you prefer less spicy.

Hummus

Ingredients

1 ½ c Chickpeas
¼ c Tahini
1 clove Garlic
½ t Cumin

2 T Extra Virgin Olive Oil
¼ c Lemon Juice
1/8 t Sea Salt

Directions

Mix ingredients in a blender or food processor.

Hummus & Veggie Wrap

Ingredients
1 Whole Wheat Tortilla
¼ c Hummus
2 Leaves Romain Lettuce
¼ Avocado, chopped
¼ Cucumber, chopped
¼ Red Bell Pepper, chopped

Directions
1. Lay the tortilla flat and spread the hummus in the center of each tortilla.
2. Layer the romaine leaves, avocado, cucumber, and bell pepper. Roll the tortilla tightly while folding the ends in.

Indian Vegetable Curry

Serving Size: 6

Ingredients:
1 T Light Sesame Oil
1 c Onion
2 cloves Fresh Garlic
1 t Ground Cumin
1 t Sea Salt
1 t Black Pepper
1 T Curry Powder
2 T Fresh Ginger
2 T Whole Wheat Flour
2 c Water
1 c Broccoli Florets
1 c Cauliflower Florets
½ c Carrots
½ c Fresh or Frozen Green Peas
½ Apple
½ c Raisins
1 c Firm Tofu or 1 cup cooked beans

Directions:
1. Peel and chop the carrots. Dice the apple and onion. Cube the tofu. Chop/mince the garlic. Grate the ginger.
2. Heat oil in a large skillet and sauté the onion and garlic until golden. Be careful not to burn the garlic. Add the cumin, salt, pepper, curry, and ginger and stir.
3. Mix in the flour and cook for 2-3 minutes. Slowly add water and mix until creamy and smooth.
4. Add the broccoli, cauliflower, carrots, peas, apple, raisins, and tofu. Cook until the mixture is thick and bubbly and the vegetables are tender.

Israelite Unleavened Bread with Olive Oil Dipping Sauce

Ingredients

½ c Whole Wheat Flour
3 ½ T Cold Water
4 T Extra Virgin Olive Oil
⅓ t Sea Salt

⅛ Sweet Onion
2 cloves Fresh Garlic
½ t Italian Seasoning

Directions

1. Preheat oven to 500°.
2. Chop the onion fine. Chop/mince the garlic.
3. Combine flour, water, 1 ¾ t olive oil, ¼ t salt, onion, and ½ clove garlic to form a dough and knead for 3 minutes.
4. Divide the dough into 8 balls. Flatten each ball into a thin round and prick with a fork and bake on a greased cookie sheet for 10 minutes.
5. Mix remaining olive oil, garlic, and the Italian seasoning to make dipping sauce.

Italian Vegetable Soup

Ingredients

½ c Sweet Onion
2 stalks Celery
½ c Baby Carrots
1 clove Garlic
1 c Diced Tomatoes
1 c Tomato Sauce
1 c cooked Red Kidney Beans
1 c Vegetable Broth

1 ½ t Dried Parsley
½ t Sea Salt
¼ t Oregano
¼ t Dried Basil
⅛ t Black Pepper
1 c Green Cabbage (shredded)
½ c Green Beans

Directions

1. Chop onion, celery, and carrot. Chop/mince garlic.
2. Add all ingredients into a large pot except the cabbage and green beans. Bring to a boil, reduce heat, and simmer for 20 minutes.
3. Add the cabbage and green beans. Return to a boil, then reduce and simmer until vegetables are tender (about 20-30 minutes).

Note: Quadruple recipe for leftovers. This recipe freezes great.

Kale Slaw with Fruit Slices

Ingredients

3 c Baby Kale
1 Carrot
½ c Orange Juice
½ c Lemon Juice
½ Red Onion
Salt & Pepper to taste

1 T Extra Virgin Olive Oil
1 T Vegan Mayonnaise
(or 1 T Olive Oil & 1 t Lemon Juice)
1 Naval Orange, peeled
1 Apple

Directions

1. Peel and chop the carrot. Slice the onion, orange, and apple.
2. Place kale into a salad bowl. Toss with carrot, orange juice, lemon juice, and salt. Using your hands, rube the juice into the kale and let it sit a few minutes.
3. Prepare a large bowl of ice water and a saucepan with boiling water.
4. Place the thinly sliced onion into the boiling water for 15-30 seconds. Scoop the onions out and dump them into the cold water.
5. Drain the water and blot the onions with a paper towel.
6. Add the onion, olive oil, salt, and pepper to the kale and toss well.
7. Add mayonnaise and mix. Refrigerate until ready to serve.
8. Garnish with the fruit slices.

Krunch Kale Krisps

Ingredients

6 c Kale Leaves
1 T Apple Cider Vinegar

2 T Extra Virgin Olive Oil
½ t Sea Salt

Directions

1. Preheat the oven to 350°.
2. Cut the kale leaves into 2-3" pieces.
3. Combine the vinegar, oil, and salt in a large bowl.
4. Add the kale to the mixture and toss by hand to make sure all leaves are covered.
5. Place the leaves in a single layer on a baking sheet. Bake for 20 minutes.
6. Check the kale. If not crisp, return to the oven and check in 5-minute increments. Remove when all leaves are crispy.

Lentil Salad

Ingredients

1 lb Lentils
5 c Water
2 t Sea Salt
¼ c Extra Virgin Olive Oil
1 Sweet Onion
1 Stalk Celery

⅓ Green Bell Pepper, chopped
⅓ Red Bell Pepper, chopped
¼ Pimento, optional
½ c Extra Virgin Olive Oil
2 T White Wine Vinegar
1 ½ t Sea Salt & Black Pepper

Directions

1. Boil the lentils in water with salt. Reduce heat and simmer, covered tightly for 30 minutes. Lentils should be tender, but firm.
2. Chop onion, celery, green pepper, red pepper, and pimentos.
3. Drain the lentils, toss with ½ c olive oil, and cool.
4. Add the vegetables to the lentils and mix.
5. Use remaining olive oil, white wine vinegar, and salt and pepper as dressing. Toss over salad and mix well.

Lentil Soup

The perfect detox soup.

Ingredients

½ c Pearl Barley
1 ¼ T Extra Virgin Olive Oil
½ c chopped Celery
½ c Sweet Onion
3 ¾ c Water
½ c Lentils

5 c Canned Chopped Tomatoes
1 t Sea Salt
⅛ t Ground Black Pepper
⅓ t Dried Rosemary
1 Fresh Garlic
1 Long Carrot Or ½ Cup Baby Carrots

Directions

1. Soak the barley overnight in water, then drain.
2. Chop the celery and onion. Chop/mince the garlic. Peel and shred the carrot.
3. Heat the oil in a skillet and sauté the oil, celery, and onion until tender.
4. Add the water and dry lentils.
5. Cook for 20 minutes.
6. Add the tomatoes, barley, salt, pepper, rosemary, and garlic and simmer 10 minutes.
7. Add the carrots and cook 5 more minutes.

Marinated Vegetable Salad

Ingredients

⅓ c Olive Oil
½ c Apple Cider Vinegar
1 ½ T Lemon Juice
⅓ t Ground Black Pepper
⅔ stalk Green Onion
⅔ clove Fresh Garlic

2 t Sea Salt
⅓ t Oregano
⅓ t Dry Mustard
2 small Zucchinis
2 small Summer Squash

Directions

1. Chop the green onion, zucchini, and squash. Chop/mince the garlic.
2. Mix the oil, vinegar, lemon juice, pepper, green onion, garlic, salt, oregano, and mustard. Shake well and pour over the vegetables.
3. Marinate for several hours. Stir and serve at room temperature or chilled.

Mexican Bean Salad

Serving Size: 4

Ingredients:

1 T Olive Oil
1-2 Jalapeno Peppers, optional
2 cloves Fresh Garlic
½ Yellow Onion
1 t Sea Salt
1 t Black Pepper
½ Green Bell Pepper
1 cup Diced Tomatoes

½ t Cayenne
1 t Chili Powder
¼ c Cilantro
1 c cooked Black Beans
1 c cooked Kidney Beans
1 c cooked Pinto Beans
¼ c Red Wine Vinegar or Lemon Juice

Directions:

1. Finely dice the jalapeno peppers. Dice the onion and bell pepper. Chop/mince the garlic. Chop the cilantro.
2. Heat oil in a medium skillet and sauté jalapeno and green pepper, garlic, onion, salt, and black pepper until the onion is translucent.
3. Stir in the diced green pepper, tomatoes, cayenne, chili powder, and cilantro, and heat just until cilantro begins to wilt.
4. Turn tomato and pepper mixture into a medium mixing bowl. Add all of the beans and the vinegar (or lemon juice). Mix well and chill thoroughly before serving.
5. Serve on a bed of field greens or green leafy lettuce.

Mideast Pilaf

Ingredients

6 c cooked Brown Rice
2 t Extra Virgin Olive Oil
2 Sweet Onion
⅔ c Cashews
1 ⅓ c Dried Cranberries or Raisins
2 c Dried Apricots
½ t Salt & Pepper
½ t Cinnamon
½ t Turmeric
¼ t Cardamom
¼ t Ground Cloves
⅔ c Apple Juice

Directions

1. Chop the sweet onion and apricots.
2. Heat the oil in a large skillet and sauté the onion for 3-5 minutes.
3. Add the nuts and dried fruit and cook for 2-3 minutes, or until the nuts begin to brown and the fruit is plump.
4. Add the rice, dried fruit, and spices. Stir in the apple juice.
5. Serve immediately or cold.

Moroccan Vegetable Stew

Servings: 8 servings (3 quarts)

Don't let the spices steer you away – absolutely delicious.

Ingredients:

1 large Onion
1 T Olive Oil
2 t Ground Cinnamon
2 t Ground Cumin
1 t Ground Coriander
½ t Cayenne Pepper
½ t Ground Allspice
¼ t Salt

3 c Water
1 sm. Butternut Squash
2 med. Potatoes
4 med. Carrots
3 Plum Tomatoes
2 sm. Zucchini
2 c Garbanzo Beans or Chickpeas

Directions:

1. Chop the onion and tomatoes. Peel and cube the squash and potatoes. Peel and slice the carrots. Cut the zucchini into 1-inch pieces.
2. In a large cooking pot, sauté onion in oil until tender. Add spices and salt; cook 1 minute longer.
3. Stir in the water, squash, potatoes, carrots. and tomatoes. Bring to a boil.
4. Reduce heat and simmer, uncovered, for 15-20 minutes or until the potatoes and squash are almost tender.
5. Add the zucchini and chickpeas and return to a boil. Reduce the heat and simmer, uncovered, for 5-8 minutes or until the vegetables are tender.

Moroccan Vegetarian Stew

Ingredients

¼ Sweet Onion
¾ t Extra Virgin Olive Oil
½ t Cinnamon
¼ t Cumin
¼ t Ground Coriander
⅛ t Cayenne Pepper
⅛ t Ground Allspice

1/8 t Sea Salt
¾ c Water
¼ Butternut Squash
1 sm. Red Potato
1 Carrot
½ Zucchini
½ c cooked Chickpeas

Directions

1. Dice the onion. Peel and cube the squash, potato, and carrot. Cube the zucchini.
2. Put the oil in a large cooking pot and sauté the onion until tender.
3. Add the spices and salt and cook 1 minute longer.
4. Stir in the water, squash, potato, carrot, and zucchini. Bring to a boil.
5. Reduce the heat and simmer uncovered for 15-20 minutes. (Potatoes and squash should be tender.)
6. Add the zucchini and chickpeas and return to a boil.
7. Reduce the heat and simmer uncovered for 5-8 minutes.

Muesli Mix

Ingredients

2 c Oats
1 c Pecans (or other nut)
1 oz Coconut, Unsweetened Shredded
⅓ c Sesame Seeds

⅓ c Whole Flax seeds
2 T Cinnamon
1 c Blueberries
1 c Pitted Dates

Directions

Mix all ingredients and store in an air-tight container.

Nutty Veggie Burger with Mango Salsa

Ingredients

½ c Walnuts
½ c Sweet Onion (Diced)
½ c Mushrooms
1 ½ t Sea Salt & Black Pepper
2 c cooked Black Beans
(or Garbanzos, Pintos, Lentils)
2 T Tahini
1 T Extra Virgin Olive Oil
½ c Sunflower Seeds
1 c cooked Brown Rice

Salsa
2 Mangoes, chopped
1 c Red Bell Pepper, diced finely
4 fl oz Pineapple Juice
½ c Lime Juice
¼ t Ground Cumin
1 T Cilantro (Chopped)
½ t Sea Salt & Black Pepper

Directions

1. Toast the walnuts at 375° for 8-10 minutes. Cool and chop finely.
2. Dice the onion, mushrooms, and salt/pepper.
3. Puree the beans and tahini in a blender until smooth, adding water as needed.
4. In a medium skillet, heat the olive oil and sauté the onions and mushrooms with ¾ t of salt and pepper until the mushrooms are limp. Remove from heat and allow to cool.
5. Combine the bean mixture and mushroom mixture in a medium mixing bowl.
6. Stir in walnuts and sunflower seeds.
7. Add rice and stir.
8. Chill for 1-2 hours.
9. Shape mixture into burger patties, about 3-4" wide.
10. Sauté, grill, or broil about 5 minutes per side. Serve topped with Mango Salsa.
11. For salsa: Mix mango, red bell pepper, lime juice, cumin, cilantro and salt/pepper. Refrigerate for up to 4 days.

Oatmeal with Blueberries

Ingredients

1 c Water
½ c Old Fashioned or Freshly Flaked Oats
½ c Blueberries
Pinch of salt

Directions

1. Bring the water and oats to a boil in a small saucepan. Reduce to a steady simmer and cook for about 5 minutes, stirring occasionally. Oats should be tender and most of the water will be absorbed.
2. Transfer the cooked oats into a bowl and top with blueberries.

Oven Roasted Broccoli & Cauliflower

Ingredients

3 c Broccoli Florets
3 c Cauliflower Florets
2 ½ T Extra Virgin Olive Oil
½ t Sea Salt

¼ t Ground Black Pepper
2 cloves Fresh Garlic
¾ t Red Pepper Flakes

Directions

1. Heat the oven to 350°.
2. Chop/mince the garlic.
3. Toss the broccoli and cauliflower in a large bowl with the olive oil, salt, and black pepper.
4. Add the garlic and red pepper flakes and toss well to coat thoroughly.
5. Coat a shallow baking pan with cooking spray or coconut oil and arrange the vegetables in a single layer.
6. Roast for 10-15 minutes, stirring halfway through. Vegetables are ready when they are slightly tender and beginning to brown.

Overnight Oatmeal with Fruit

Ingredients

2 c Oats
4 ½ c Water
1 t Sea Salt
1 T Coconut Oil

1 Apple, diced
¼ c Raisins
¼ c Pitted Dates
1 t Cinnamon

Directions

1. Grease crockpot.
2. Combine oats, water, salt, and coconut oil in the crockpot.
3. Cook on low for 8 hours.
4. Scoop the desired amount of cooked oats and add diced fruit and cinnamon.

Pancakes with Fruit Sauce

Ingredients

1 c Kamut Flour	½ c Strawberries
½ t Sea Salt	½ c Raspberries
1 Banana	¼ c Water
2 T Extra Virgin Olive Oil	¼ t Stevia
½ c Blueberries	¼ t Sea Salt

Directions

1. Wash berries and slice strawberries.
2. Put berries and water in a small pot. Cook over medium high heat until thickened. Add stevia and salt and stir well.
3. Mix dry ingredients. Add banana and olive oil.
4. Drop onto hot skillet in spoonfuls and cook for about 2 minutes on each side. Serve with warm fruit sauce.

Peruvian Quinoa Stew

Serving Size: 4

Ingredients:

½ c Quinoa	2 Tomatoes
1 c Water	1 c Water or Vegetable Stock
2 Onions	2 t Ground Cumin
2 cloves Fresh Garlic	½ t Chili Powder
1 T Vegetable Oil	1 t Ground Coriander
1 stalk Celery	Cayenne to taste
1 Carrot	1 t Oregano
1 Bell Pepper	Fresh Cilantro
1 Zucchini	

Directions:

1. Chop the onions and cilantro. Chop/mince the garlic. Peel the carrot and cut on the diagonal into ¼" thick slices. Slice the celery and bell pepper. Cube the zucchini. Dice the tomatoes.
2. Place quinoa and 1 cup of water in a pot and cook covered on medium-low heat for about 15 minutes, until soft.
3. While the quinoa is cooking, place the onions, garlic, and vegetable oil in a covered soup pot and sauté on medium heat for 5 minutes.
4. Add the celery and carrots to the soup pot and cook an additional 5 minutes, stirring often.
5. Add the bell pepper, zucchini, tomatoes, and 1 cup of water or vegetable stock to pot. Stir in cumin, chili powder, coriander, cayenne, and oregano to soup pot. Simmer covered for 10 to 15 minutes until vegetables are tender.
6. Stir in cooked quinoa and salt to taste.
7. Top with chopped cilantro. Serve immediately.

Pine-Orange-Banana Smoothie

Serving Size: 1

Ingredients:

1 Banana

½ c Orange Juice

½ c Pineapple chunks

Directions:

1. Cut the pineapple into bite-sized pieces. Peel and break the banana in 2-3 pieces.
2. Blend all ingredients until smooth.
3. For a frozen smoothie, add ice cubes.

Popeye Burgers

Ingredients

1 box Frozen Spinach, thawed

1 Russet Potato

1 Sweet Onion

1 T Garlic Powder

1 T Dried Onion Flakes

½ t Paprika

½ c Tomato Sauce

½ c Whole Wheat Matzo

½ c Oats

½ c Cornmeal

1 t Seasoned Salt

1 T Dijon Mustard

1 T Extra Virgin Olive Oil

Directions

1. Peel and grate the potato. Chop the onion finely. Chop/mince the garlic. Crush the matzo.
2. Blend all of the ingredients thoroughly in a large mixing bowl, adding a little more cornmeal if the mixture is too wet, or water if the mixture is too dry.
3. Form the mixture into thin patties and fry in a lightly oiled, nonstick pan over medium heat.

Uncooked patties may be frozen.

Frozen spinach may need to be squeezed with a paper towel to remove moisture.

Quick & Easy Breakfast Bar

Ingredients

3 c Oats
1 c Whole Wheat Flour
1 c Chocolate Protein Powder
1 t Baking Powder
1 t Baking Soda
¼ t Nutmeg
½ t Cinnamon
1 ¼ c Unsweetened Applesauce
1 t Vanilla Extract

Directions

1. Mix all ingredients. If too dry, add more applesauce.
2. Spread the mixture in an 8 x 13 baking dish.
3. Bake at 300° for 20 minutes.

Quinoa Pilaf

Ingredients

6 cups Water
3 c Quinoa
2 T Extra Virgin Olive Oil
1 clove Fresh Garlic
2 Carrot
4 Green Onions
½ Stalk Celery
¼ Green Bell Pepper
¼ Red Bell Pepper
¼ c Mushrooms
⅛ t. Oregano
½ c Sliced Almonds

Directions

1. Bring 6 cups of water to boil. Add quinoa and simmer covered for 25-30 minutes.
2. Dice carrot, green onions, celery, green bell pepper, red bell pepper, and mushrooms. Chop/mince garlic.
3. Sauté vegetables and garlic in olive oil until tender.
4. Add oregano and stir.
5. Add vegetables to quinoa. Sprinkle with salt and stir.
6. Roast the almonds in a skillet until lightly golden brown and add to mix.

Rice with Steamed Vegetables

Ingredients

2 c cooked Brown Rice
1 Butternut Squash, peeled
1 Zucchini
¼ Green Cabbage
1 c Broccoli
Salt, Pepper to taste
1 t Apple Cider Vinegar

Directions

1. Dice the vegetables and steam until they reach desired softness.
   To steam, is to cook in a double boiler or in a cooking dish over hot boiling water. Another option is to stir fry in water in a skillet.
2. Mix the rice and vegetables together and season with salt, pepper, or apple cider vinegar.

Roasted Broccoli

Ingredients

1 ½ c Broccoli
1 ⅛ t Avocado Oil
⅛ t Garlic Powder
Dash Sea Salt

Directions

1. Preheat the oven to 400°.
2. Line a baking sheet with parchment paper.
3. Cut the florets into bite-sized pieces and arrange on the baking sheet. Season with the avocado oil, garlic powder, and sea salt. Toss well and bake for 20 minutes, tossing halfway through. Check for doneness.

Savory Stuffed Peppers

Ingredients

2 c cooked Brown Rice
2 c cooked Black Beans, drained
1 T Olive Oil
1 Sweet Onion
1 T Chili Powder
½ t Cumin
¼ t Paprika
½ t Sea Salt

¼ t Ground Black Pepper
1 t Cayenne Pepper
½ c Carrot
¾ c Mushrooms, including stems
4 Green Bell Peppers
2 c Salsa
1 ½ T Cilantro
1 Avocado

Directions

1. Preheat the oven to 400°.
2. Finely chop the onion and mushrooms.
3. Peel and shred the carrot.
4. Halve and seed the bell peppers.
5. Lightly coat the peppers with olive oil and roast in a baking dish in the pre-heated oven for 20-25 minutes.
6. Remove the peppers from the oven and cool.
7. In a bowl, mix all seasonings, onion, black beans, corn, carrots, mushrooms, and rice. Stir. Add salsa and mix well.
8. Spoon the rice mixture into each half of the bell peppers and place back onto the baking dish.
9. Cook for 15-20 minutes.
10. Remove from the oven and top with cilantro and avocado slices.

Spanish Paella

Ingredients

½ c Brown Rice
2 c Vegetable Broth (or water)
½ c Basmati Rice
1 T Extra Virgin Olive Oil
1 Yellow Onion
2 Garlic Cloves
1 Red Bell Pepper
1 Green Bell Pepper
½ c Mushrooms
1 ½ c Eggplant
½ c Black Olives
1 t Sea Salt
½ t Ground Black Pepper
½ t Cumin
½ t Saffron
2 c Diced Tomatoes

Directions

1. Combine the brown rice and vegetable broth in a large saucepan and bring to a boil. Reduce heat to simmer and cook covered for about 10 minutes.
2. Add the basmati rice and cook for 30 minutes.
3. Preheat the oven to 400°.
4. Chop the onion, bell peppers, mushrooms, eggplant, and olives. Chop/mince the garlic.
5. Heat the oil in a large, oven-proof skillet. Add the onion, garlic, red and green pepper, mushrooms, eggplant, olives, salt, pepper, saffron, and cumin. Sauté until the peppers are tender (about 5 minutes).
6. Stir the tomatoes and rice mixture into the vegetables and bake for 10 minutes, or until heated through and bubbly.

Spelt Chapatti

Ingredients

½ c Water
3 T Extra Virgin Olive Oil
½ t Sea Salt
2 c Spelt Flour
1 t Italian Seasoning

Directions

1. Preheat oven to 375°.
2. Combine the water, 1 T oil, and salt in a large mixing bowl.
3. Add flour gradually, stirring until the mixture is thick. Continue to add flour, working the dough by hand until a soft ball forms. Knead until smooth.
4. Let the dough rest, covered, for 10-20 minutes.
5. Form the dough into 2" balls. Flatten into 5" circles.
6. Place on oiled baking sheet and bake for 2-3 minutes. Flip and bake an additional 2-3 minutes.
7. Mix remaining 2 T of olive oil and Italian Seasoning to make dipping oil.

Steamed Vegetables with Quinoa

Ingredients

4 c cooked Quinoa
2 c Broccoli
1 Red Bell Pepper
4 Carrots
¼ c Olive Oil

Directions

1. Steam vegetables to desired tenderness (5-10 minutes).
2. Stir olive oil into cooked quinoa and add steamed vegetables.

Surprise Delight Juice

Ingredients

1 c Pineapple, crushed or chopped
1 c Coconut Water

Directions

1. Blend ingredients.
2. Add a dash of stevia if desired.

Surprise Delight Smoothie

Servings: 1

Recipe: The Antioxidant Diet; Robin Jeep and Dr. Couey

Ingredients:

1 c Unsweetened Pineapple Juice
1 c Water
1 c Frozen Pineapple Chunks
1/6 Cantaloupe
1 Carrot
4 Kale Leaves
1 Kiwi
1 T Freshly Ground Flaxseed

Directions:

1. Cube the cantaloupe. Strip the kale leaves from the stems. Peel and slice the kiwi.
2. Combine in a blender and blend until smooth.

Sweet Brown Rice with Spicy Sauce

Ingredients

4 c cooked Brown Rice
1 t Extra Virgin Olive Oil
1 Yellow Onion
3 clove Fresh Garlic
2 T Ground Ginger

⅓ c Water
2 T Bragg's Liquid Aminos
½ t Chili Sauce
2 t Sesame Oil
¼ c Chopped Fresh Cilantro

Directions

1. Cook the brown rice following instructions.
2. Heat olive oil in a large skillet and sauté onion, garlic, and ginger for 2 minutes.
3. Add all other ingredients except (½ the cilantro) and stir until blended. Cover and cook on medium heat 5-7 minutes (until all ingredients are heated through).
4. Garnish with remaining cilantro.

Sweet Potato Pie

Ingredients

4 Sweet Potatoes
1 ½ c Broccoli
1 c Collard Greens
¼ Head Cauliflower
4 oz Mushrooms
3 Garlic Cloves
½ Red Bell Pepper
1 ¼ c Vegetable Broth

1 ½ t Chili Powder
1 ½ T Tomato Paste
1 t Bragg's Liquid Aminos
1 T Cashew Butter
1 ½ c cooked Red Kidney Beans
¼ c Pecans
1 ½ c Mixed Greens

Directions

1. Wash the potatoes, prick with a fork, wrap in foil, and bake at 350° for 1 hour.
2. Let the potatoes cool.
3. Chop the broccoli, collard greens, cauliflower, mushrooms, bell pepper, and pecans. Chop/mince the garlic.
4. In a large pot, combine the broccoli, collard greens, cauliflower, mushrooms, and bell peppers in the vegetable broth. Simmer covered for 15 minutes.
5. Add the chili powder, tomato paste, and liquid aminos. Cook until almost tender (about 10 minutes).
6. Peel and smash the sweet potatoes.
7. Add the cashew butter and beans to the vegetable mixture and stir well.
8. Spread the mixture in a baking dish. Top with the mashed sweet potatoes.
9. Sprinkle with chili powder and chopped pecans.
10. Bake for 20-30 minutes, until hot and pecans are light brown.
11. Serve hot or cold, alone or over mixed greens.

Tabouli (Stuffed in Tomatoes)

Ingredients

1 c Bulgur Wheat
1 ½ c Water
⅓ c Olive Oil
¼ c Lemon Juice
2 t Sea Salt
½ t Garlic Powder
1 t Oregano
⅛ t Ground Allspice
2 Cucumber
1 c Parsley
½ c Mint Leaves
4 Tomatoes

Directions

1. Bring the water to a boil and pour over the wheat. Let sit 30 minutes.
2. Chop/mince the garlic. Peel, seed, and dice the cucumber. Chop the parsley and mint.
3. Slice one tomato in half and core it. Dice the other tomato.
4. Combine the oil, lemon juice, garlic powder, oregano, and all the spices and mix well.
5. Add to the wheat, vegetables, parsley, and mint and mix well.
6. Stuff the tomato halves with the mixture.

Taco Soup

Ingredients

4 c Water
2 c Bulgur Wheat
2 Sweet Onions
2 c Frozen Corn
14 oz. can Diced Tomatoes
1 can Black Olives
2 cans Pinto Beans
1 c Mexican Tomatoes
1 can Tomatoes with Chiles
½ c chopped Green Olives
1 ½ t Sea Salt
2 t Parsley

Directions

1. Bring 4 cups of water to a boil, then stir in Bulgur wheat and reduce to simmer.
2. Once bulgur has absorbed water (about 15 minutes), add all other ingredients. Heat through.
3. Can add more liquid, if desired.

Tex Mex Chili

Ingredients

¼ c Extra Virgin Olive Oil
3 c Sweet Onion
12 Cloves Garlic
2 Jalapeno Peppers
2 T Cumin
1 ⅓ T Oregano
1 t Cinnamon
2 T Ground Coriander
2 T Chili Powder

1 t Ground Black Pepper
1 t Sea Salt
4 c cooked Black Beans
4 c Stewed Tomatoes
4 c Corn
1 oz Dark Chocolate Powder or 2 ounces Dark Chocolate 70% or higher cacoa
2 T Lime Juice
2T Bragg's Liquid Aminos

Directions

1. Chop the onion and jalapeno. Chop/mince the garlic.
2. Heat a pan with olive oil and sauté the onion and garlic until soft and starting to caramelize.
3. Add the spices, jalapenos, and stewed tomatoes. Simmer for 5 minutes.
4. Using an immersion blender, grind this mixture to smooth.
5. Add beans, corn, chocolate, lime juice, and liquid aminos. Simmer for 20 minutes.

Three Bean Soup

Servings: 6

Ingredients:

1 T Olive Oil
1 c Onion
3 cloves Fresh Garlic
1 t Dried Rosemary Leaves
¼ t Dried Thyme Leaves
2 Bay Leaves
1 Whole Clove
¼ t Pepper
5 c Vegetable Broth
1½ c cooked Baby Lima Beans (or navy beans)
1½ c cooked Chickpeas
1½ c cooked Red Beans
3 T Tomato Paste
1½ c cooked barley or rice
1 lg. Potato
1 c Carrots
1 c packed Spinach Leaves

Directions:

1. Chop the onion and spinach. Chop/mince the garlic. Dice the potato and slice the carrots.
2. Heat oil in a large soup pot over medium heat; sauté onions, and garlic for 2-3 minutes or until onions are tender.
3. Add vegetable broth, beans, spices and tomato paste to pot; heat to boiling, stirring to prevent sticking.
4. Reduce heat and simmer, uncovered, for 10-15 minutes.
5. Add barley, potato, carrots, and spinach and simmer 10 more minutes until all ingredients are well heated and tender. Discard bay leaves and clove before serving.

Three-Bean Indian Dal with Green Salad

Ingredients

2 T Olive Oil
¾ c Red Onion
2 stalks Celery
4 cloves Fresh Garlic
1 Green Bell Pepper
1 t Sea Salt
½ t White Pepper
1 T Celery Seed
1 T Cumin
2 t Coriander

2 T Ground Ginger
2 Tomatoes
3 c Water
1 c Lentils
1 c cooked Black Beans
1 c cooked Chickpeas
¼ c Fresh Cilantro, chopped
6 c Mixed Greens
⅓ c Olive Oil
⅓ c Apple Cider Vinegar

Directions

1. Dice red onion, celery, green bell pepper, and tomato. Chop/mince garlic.
2. Heat oil in a large pot and sauté onion, celery, garlic, green pepper, salt, and white pepper until veggies are tender.
3. Add celery seed, cumin, coriander, and ginger and sauté for 3 minutes.
4. Add tomatoes and sauté until soft and juicy.
5. Add water, lentils, black beans, chickpeas, and cilantro. Cover and simmer for 15 minutes. Serve hot, garnished with cilantro.
6. Wash and chop greens and drizzle with olive oil and vinegar.

Toasted Almond Granola

Servings: 8 cups

Ingredients:

4 c Oats
1 c slivered Raw Almonds
1 c whole Raw Almonds
½ c Unsweetened Shredded Coconut
1 t Cinnamon

½ t Sea Salt
3 T coconut oil
¼ c Olive Oil
1 T Stevia
1 t Pure Vanilla Extract

Directions:

1. Place a rack in the upper third and middle of the oven and preheat to 325°.
2. Line one large or two small baking sheets with parchment paper and set aside.
3. Stir together the oats, whole almonds, slivered almonds, unsweetened coconut, cinnamon, and salt. Set aside.
4. In a medium saucepan, melt together coconut oil, oil, and stevia until the mixture begins to boil. Carefully stir together until well mixed. Add the vanilla extract.
5. Pour the warm mixture over the oat and almond mixture and toss together with a wooden spoon, ensuring that all of the oat mixture gets moistened by the oil mixture.
6. Spread mixture onto a prepared baking sheet(s) and bake for 25-30 minutes. Stir the mixture twice during baking.
7. Remove from the oven, let cool, and store in an airtight container for up to two weeks.

Toasted Walnuts

Ingredients

Walnuts

Directions

1. Preheat oven to 350°.
2. Prepare a baking sheet with parchment paper and spread the walnuts out in one layer.
3. Toast for 5 minutes, flip the walnuts, and toast for 5 additional minutes.

Tomato Walnut Salad

Ingredients:

3 Tomatoes
2 Green Bell Peppers
½ c Walnuts
¼ c Fresh Parsley
Extra Virgin Olive Oil to taste
Salt and Pepper to taste

Directions:

1. Chop the tomatoes, walnuts, and parsley. Seed and chop the peppers.
2. In a salad bowl, toss together the tomatoes, peppers, walnuts, parsley, olive oil and salt and pepper to taste.

Turkish Salad

Ingredients

1 head Green Lettuce
1 Green Bell Pepper
1 Red Bell Pepper
½ Cucumber
½ Red Onion
2 c Diced Tomatoes
3 T Extra Virgin Olive Oil
3 T Lemon Juice
1 Garlic Clove
1 T Fresh Parsley
1 T Mint Leaves
½ t Sea Salt
⅓ t Black Pepper
1 c Black Olives, chopped

Directions

1. Chop lettuce, green bell pepper, red bell pepper, cucumber, red onion, parsley, and mint. Chop/mince garlic.
2. Place lettuce, peppers, cucumber, tomatoes, and onion in a large serving bowl.
3. In a separate bowl, whisk olive oil, lemon juice, garlic, parsley, mint, salt, and pepper. Pour over salad and toss.
4. Top with olives.

Tuscan Villa Bean Soup

Ingredients

1 t Extra Virgin Olive Oil
1 c Sweet Onion (chopped)
½ c Celery (chopped)
3 cloves Fresh Garlic
1 T Whole Wheat Flour
1 t Dried Rosemary
¼ t Thyme
2 Bay Leaf
1 Whole Cloves

¼ t Ground Black Pepper
5 c Vegetable Broth
1 ½ c White Beans (cooked)
1 ½ c Chickpeas, cooked
⅓ c Organic Ketchup
1 Red Potato
1 c Carrot (sliced)
1 ½ c Barley, cooked

Directions

1. Dice onion and celery. Dice/mince garlic.
2. Heat oil in a large soup pot over medium heat and sauté onions, celery, and garlic for 2-3 minutes or until onions are tender.
3. Stir in the flour and seasonings.
4. Add vegetable broth, beans, and ketchup. Heat to boiling, stirring frequently to prevent sticking. Reduce heat and simmer uncovered for 10-15 minutes.
5. Add barley, potato, and carrot. Simmer 10 minutes until all ingredients are tender and heated through.
6. Discard bay leaf and clove before serving.

Vegetable Fried Rice

Ingredients

2 c cooked Brown Rice
1 T Extra Virgin Olive Oil
1 c Asparagus
2 Red Bell Peppers
8 Scallions

2 Fresh Garlic Cloves
2 T Ground Ginger
2 T Bragg's Liquid Aminos
¼ c Rice Vinegar
2 t Toasted Sesame Oil

Directions

1. Cut asparagus into 1" pieces, thinly slice bell pepper into 1" pieces, and chop/mince garlic.
2. Coat a large nonstick wok or skillet with oil and turn on medium heat.
3. Add bell pepper, scallions, garlic, and ginger to the pan. Cook, stirring, until vegetables are tender.
4. Add cooked rice, liquid aminos, and vinegar. Cook until the liquid is absorbed.
5. Remove from the heat and stir in the sesame oil. Add hot sauce or red pepper flakes if desired.

Vegetable Pizza

Ingredients

1 c Whole Wheat Flour
⅓ c Cold Water
2 T Olive Oil
1 t Sea Salt
¼ Sweet Onion
2 cloves Fresh Garlic
2 T Tomato Paste

½ c Tomato Sauce
Dash Ground Black Pepper
¼ t Oregano
3 Mushrooms
¼ c Broccoli
¼ Red Bell Pepper

Directions

1. Preheat the oven to 500°.
2. Chop the onion and chop/mince garlic.
3. Combine the flour, water, 1 T. olive oil, ½ t salt, onion, and 1 minced clove of garlic to form dough. Knead for 3 minutes.
4. Divide dough into 4 balls. Flatten each into a thin round and prick each with a fork. Bake for 5 minutes.
5. Combine the remaining garlic, ½ t salt, tomato paste, tomato sauce, ground black pepper, oregano, and remaining olive oil. Spread onto the dough.
6. Wash and chop desired vegetables. Bake 5-10 minutes until heated through.

Vegetable Pizza 2

Recipe: The Antioxidant Diet; Robin Jeep & Dr. Couey

Ingredients:

2 c Broccoli
1 lg. Red Bell Pepper
1 c Mushrooms
1 clove Fresh Garlic
½ t Bragg's Liquid Aminos
1 T Balsamic Vinegar
1 t Italian Seasoning
½ c Pasta Sauce
2 Ezekiel Sprouted Grain Tortillas
4 oz Non-Dairy Cheese, grated
5 oz Fresh Spinach

Directions:

1. Chop the broccoli, pepper, mushrooms, and spinach. Chop/mince the garlic.
2. Preheat oven to 350°.
3. In a large bowl, toss broccoli, bell peppers, and mushrooms with garlic, liquid aminos, vinegar, and seasoning mix.
4. Roast vegetables on a lightly oiled cookie sheet, turning occasionally, and mounding to keep from drying out, for 30 minutes.
5. Remove vegetables when done and raise oven temperature to 450°.
6. Spread a thin layer of pasta sauce on tortilla, sprinkle cheese, and distribute roasted vegetables and spinach.
7. Bake on a cookie sheet for approximately 7 minutes or until cheese is melted and tortilla browns around edges.

Vegetable Soup

Ingredients

6 c Vegetable Broth
3 c Diced Tomatoes
4 Bay Leaves
1 t. Sea Salt & Black Pepper
1 t Thyme
1 t Fresh Oregano
1 Clove Garlic
1 t Red Pepper Flakes, optional
3 Yellow Potatoes
1 Sweet Onion
2 Carrots
¼ stalk Celery
2 c Frozen Green Beans
2 c Frozen Corn
1 c cooked Black Beans

Directions

1. Heat the vegetable broth, diced tomatoes, and spices over medium heat.
2. Dice the potatoes, carrots, onion, and celery. Add all the vegetables to the broth and simmer for 30-45 minutes. Add water as needed.
3. Remove the bay leaves before serving.

Vegetarian Chili

Ingredients

½ c Sweet Onion (chopped)
¼ c Green Bell Pepper
1 clove Fresh Garlic
1 ¾ T Extra Virgin Olive Oil
1 ⅛ T Chili Powder
¼ t Oregano
¼ t Cumin
¼ t Black Pepper
1 ⅛ c Zucchini (Chopped)
⅔ c Carrot (Shredded)
2 ⅔ c Diced Tomatoes
1 ¾ c cooked Red Kidney Beans
1 c cooked Chickpeas

Directions

1. Chop the onion, bell pepper, and zucchini. Chop/mince the garlic. Peel and shred the carrot.
2. Sauté the onions, peppers, and garlic in olive oil in a large pot until soft.
3. Add chili powder, oregano, cumin, black pepper, zucchini, and carrot, and stir.
4. Cook for 1 hour over low heat, stirring occasionally. Add ½ - 1 c of water if necessary.
5. Stir in tomatoes, kidney beans, and chickpeas and bring to a boil.
6. Reduce heat and simmer 10 minutes or until thick.

Veggie Medley Tomato Sauce with Spaghetti Squash

Ingredients

1 T Extra Virgin Olive Oil
½ clove Fresh Garlic
½ Sweet Onion
½ c Mushrooms
1 Carrot
½ Green Bell Pepper
1 Stalk Celery
½ t Ground Black Pepper
¼ t Sea Salt
1 lb Roma Tomatoes
2 ½ T Tomato Paste
2 T Basil Leaves
1 T Fresh Oregano, or 1 t dried
1 T Fresh Thyme or 1 t dried
1 T Fresh Rosemary or 1 t dried
1 Spaghetti Squash

Directions

1. Chop the onion, mushrooms, carrot, bell pepper, celery, and tomatoes. Finely chop the basil, oregano, thyme, and rosemary.
2. Cut the spaghetti squash in half and boil until tender. Use half for this recipe and freeze the other half for a recipe later.
3. Heat oil in a large saucepan and sauté garlic until fragrant.
4. Add the onion, mushrooms, carrots, green peppers, celery, black pepper, and salt. Cook until the carrots are tender.
5. Stir in the tomatoes, tomato paste, and herbs. Simmer about 20 minutes.
6. Use a fork to "peel" the spaghetti squash meat from the peel.
7. Serve the cooked vegetables over the spaghetti squash.

Veggie Wraps

Recipe: The Antioxidant Diet; Robin Jeep & Dr. Couey

Servings: 4

Ingredients:

1 c Lentils
½ c Celery
1 Orange
1 clove Fresh Garlic
½ T Balsamic Vinegar
3 t Olive Oil
1 T Dried Currants

¼ c Red Pepper
1 T Parsley
1 T Mint
1 t Bragg's Liquid Aminos
¼ c Walnuts
12 large leaf lettuce leaves

Directions:

1. Cook the lentils according to package instructions.
2. Chop the celery, pepper, parsley, mint, and walnuts. Chop/mince the garlic. Peel, section, chop and seed the orange.
3. Combine all ingredients except for lettuce leaves in a bowl and mix well.
4. Spread the mixture on each lettuce leaf and roll.

Verry Berry Drink

Ingredients

4 Strawberries
¼ c Raspberries
¼ c Blueberries

½ Banana, frozen is best
3 T Chocolate or Vanilla Protein Powder
½ c Apple Juice

Directions

Mix together in blender.

White Bean Dip

Ingredients

2 c cooked White Navy Beans
5 Garlic cloves
⅓ c Fresh Dill
⅓ c Mint Leaves

2 T Parsley
2 T Olive Oil
1 ½ T Lemon Juice
½ t Sea Salt

Directions

1. Soak the beans overnight in cold water.
2. Chop/mince garlic. Chop the dill, mint, and parsley.
3. Drain the beans, reserving ¼ c of liquid.
4. Process beans and reserve liquid (1/4 cup) in a blender. Add garlic, dill, mint, parsley, olive oil, lemon juice, and salt and blend.
5. Add more oil or bean liquid if needed.
6. Puree until smooth.
7. Taste and adjust for seasoning. (Add red pepper flakes or powder for added zing.)

Whole Grain Crackers

This recipe only takes about 5 minutes to mix and roll out - super easy!!

Serving Size: 8

Ingredients:

¾ c Whole Wheat Flour
½ c 7-Grain Cereal, unsweetened
½ t Sea Salt
2 T Olive Oil

¼ c Water
1 t Seasoning of choice
Chili Powder, Dried Herbs, etc.

Directions:

1. Preheat the oven to 400°.
2. Put cereal in blender to make powdery.
3. In a large bowl, combine the flour, cereal, and salt. Add the olive oil and water.
4. Using a large rubber spatula or wooden spoon, stir vigorously until dough comes together and forms a ball. If it's too sticky to handle, add flour, no more than a tablespoon at a time.
5. Place parchment paper that will fit a baking sheet on the counter. Lightly dust with flour. Roll out the dough until ⅛-inch thickness, it should be very thin!
6. Bake for 12-15 minutes or until light brown.
7. Cool for 10-15 minutes on a wire rack.
8. Break into pieces about the size of a saltine cracker. You can make additional batches while the first batch is baking. The parchment paper can be re-used for additional batches.

Wild Mushroom Cabbage Rolls

Serving Size: 8

Ingredients:

½ c Pine Nuts (or favorite nuts)
1 T Olive Oil
1 c Mushrooms
¼ c Shallots

2 cloves Fresh Garlic
1 t Sea Salt
2 c cooked Brown Rice
1 lb. Green Cabbage Leaves

Directions:

1. Chop the mushrooms and shallots. Chop/mince the garlic.
2. Heat the oven to 375°.
3. Toast pine nuts for 5 minutes.
4. Heat oil in a medium skillet and sauté mushrooms, shallots, garlic and salt until mushrooms are limp.
5. Stir in the pine nuts and brown rice and let cool.
6. Wash individual cabbage leaves, steam for 1 minute, and let cool.
7. Stack 2-3 cabbage leaves, one on top of the other, and spoon ⅛ of the rice filling onto the stacked leaves. Roll the cabbage leaves around the filling and place in an oiled casserole dish, seam side down.
8. Cover lightly with foil and bake for 20-30 minutes.

Yummy Brown Rice with Apple

Ingredients

1 c cooked Brown Rice
1 Apple, chopped
1 T Raisins
¼ t Sea Salt

½ t Cinnamon
1 t Coconut Oil
½ t Stevia

Directions

1. Preheat oven to 350°.
2. Mix all ingredients together in a small casserole dish.
3. Bake for 15 minutes.

Zesty Rice & Bean Salad

Ingredients

2 T Olive Oil
1 clove Garlic
½ t Ground Red Pepper
¼ c Lime Juice
¼ t Sea Salt
2 c cooked Brown Rice

1 ½ c cooked Black Beans
1 ½ c cooked Red Kidney Beans
4 Green Onions
¼ c Mint Leaves
¼ c Cilantro

Directions:

1. Chop/mince the garlic. Chop the green onion, mint, and cilantro.
2. Wisk together the oil, garlic, ground red pepper, lime juice, and salt.
3. Add the remaining ingredients and stir to coat.
4. Cover and chill for at least 1 hour.

Recipes

Bean Hummus	50
Better Bean Burgers	51
Black Bean and Mango Salsa	52
Black Bean Dip	52
Broccoli & Carrots	52
Butternut Squash Soup	53
Chickpea Salad	53
Classic Carrot Soup	54
Cream of Wheat w/ Almond Milk & Applesauce	54
Crispy Beans	55
Cumin Roasted Walnuts	55
Daniel Fast Black Bean Soup	56
Daniel Fast Breakfast Burrito	56
Daniel Fast Cabbage Rolls	57
Daniel Fast Cherry Berry Muesli	57
Daniel Fast Smoothie	58
Daniel Fast Sweet Potato Salad	58
Dried Fruit Balls	58
Fall Harvest Salad	59
Fast Italian Tomato-Bean Soup	59
Fruit Kabobs	60
Fruit Plate	60
Fruitful Rice Pudding	60
Green Salad with Corn Chips	61
Green Salad with Orange Slices	61
Healthy Banana Cookies	62
Healthy Tuscan White Bean Salad	62
Hot and Spicy Hummus	63
Hummus	63
Hummus & Veggie Wrap	64
Indian Vegetable Curry	64
Israelite Unleavened Bread	65
Italian Vegetable Soup	65
Kale Slaw with Fruit Slices	66
Krunch Kale Krisps	66
Lentil Salad	67
Lentil Soup	67
Marinated Vegetable Salad	68
Mexican Bean Salad	68
Mideast Pilaf	69
Moroccan Vegetable Stew	70
Moroccan Vegetarian Stew	71
Muesli Mix	71
Nutty Veggie Burger with Mango Salsa	72
Oatmeal with Blueberries	72
Oven Roasted Broccoli & Cauliflower	73
Overnight Oatmeal with Fruit	73
Pancakes with Fruit Sauce	74
Peruvian Quinoa Stew	74
Pine-Orange-Banana Smoothie	75
Popeye Burgers	75
Quick & Easy Breakfast Bar	76
Quinoa Pilaf	76
Rice with Steamed Vegetables	77
Roasted Broccoli	77
Savory Stuffed Peppers	78
Spanish Paella	79
Spelt Chapatti	79
Steamed Vegetables with Quinoa	80
Surprise Delight Juice	80
Surprise Delight Smoothie	80
Sweet Brown Rice with Spicy Sauce	81
Sweet Potato Pie	82
Tabouli (Stuffed in Tomatoes)	83
Taco Soup	83
Tex Mex Chili	84
Three Bean Soup	85
Three-Bean Indian Dal with Green Salad	86
Toasted Almond Granola	87
Toasted Walnuts	87
Tomato Walnut Salad	88
Turkish Salad	88
Tuscan Villa Bean Soup	89
Vegetable Fried Rice	89
Vegetable Pizza	90
Vegetable Pizza 2	91
Vegetable Soup	91
Vegetarian Chili	92
Veggie Medley Tomato Sauce w/ Spaghetti Squash	92
Veggie Wraps	93
Verry Berry Drink	93
White Bean Dip	94
Whole Grain Crackers	94
Wild Mushroom Cabbage Rolls	95
Yummy Brown Rice with Apple	95
Zesty Rice & Bean Salad	96